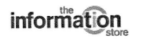
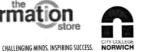

the
information store

CHALLENGING MINDS. INSPIRING SUCCESS.   **NORWICH**
CITY COLLEGE

Please return on or before the last
date stamped below.
Contact: 01603 773 114 or
01603 773 224

1 0 JAN 2014

A FINE WILL BE CHARGED FOR OVERDUE ITEMS

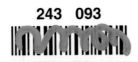

Supported by:

Asker Jeukendrup (Ed.)

Sports Nutrition
From Lab to Kitchen

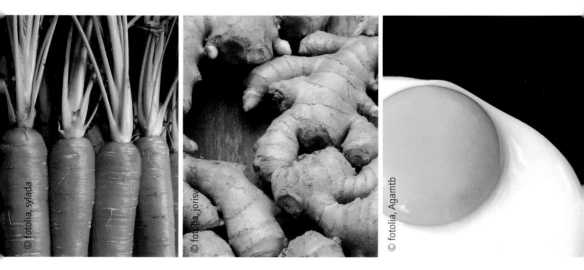

© fotolia, sylada

© fotolia, jorisv

© fotolia, Agamtb

Meyer & Meyer Sport

British Library Cataloguing in Publication Data
A catalogue record for this book is available from the British Library

Asker Jeukendrup (Ed.)
Sports Nutrition – From Lab to Kitchen
Maidenhead: Meyer & Meyer Sport (UK) Ltd., 2010
ISBN 978-1-84126-296-3

© 2010 Meyer & Meyer Sport (UK) Ltd.
Aachen, Adelaide, Auckland, Budapest, Cape Town, Graz, Indianapolis,
Maidenhead, Olten (CH), Singapore, Toronto
Member of the World
Sport Publishers' Association (WSPA)
www.w-s-p-a.org
Editing: Martha Tuninga
Printed and bound by: B.O.S.S Druck und Medien GmbH, Germany
ISBN 978-1-84126-296-3
E-Mail: info@m-m-sports.com
www.m-m-sports.com

Contents

Authors

Keith Baar
Department of Neurobiology, Physiology and Behavior, University of California, Davis, USA

Hans Braun
Sport Nutrition Department, Institute of Biochemistry, German Sport University Cologne, Germany

Elizabeth Broad
Sports Nutrition, Australian Institute of Sport, Belconnen, Australia

Louise Burke
Sports Nutrition, Australian Institute of Sport, Belconnen, Australia

Greg Cox
Sports Nutrition, Australian Institute of Sport, Belconnen, Australia

Michael Gleeson
School of Sport, Exercise and Health Sciences, Loughborough University, United Kingdom

Shona L Halson
Department of Physiology, Australian Institute of Sport, Belconnen, Australia

John Hawley
School of Medical Sciences, RMIT University, Bundoora, Australia

Asker Jeukendrup
School of Sport and Exercise Sciences, University of Birmingham, United Kingdom

Ronald Maughan
School of Sport, Exercise and Health Sciences, Loughborough University, United Kingdom

Romain Meeusen
Human Physiology & Sports Medicine, Free University Brussels, Belgium

Samuel Mettler
ETH Zurich and Swiss Federal Institute of Sport Magglingen, Switzerland

David C. Nieman
Director, Human Performance Labs, North Carolina Research Campus and Appalachian State University, Boone, NC, USA

Beate Pfeiffer
School of Sport and Exercise Sciences, University of Birmingham, United Kingdom

Stuart Phillips
Department of Kinesiology, Exercise Metabolism Research Group, McMaster University, Hamilton, ON, Canada

Brent C. Ruby
University of Montana, Montana Center for Work Physiology and Exercise Metabolism, Missoula MT, USA

Bengt Saltin
CMRC, University of Copenhagen, Denmark

Trent Stellingwerff
Nestlé Research Center, Lausanne, Switzerland

Mark Tarnopolsky
Departments of Pediatrics & Medicine, Neurometabolic & Neuromuscular Diseases, McMaster University Medical Centre, Hamilton Canada

Kevin Tipton
School of Sport and Exercise Sciences, University of Birmingham, United Kingdom

Phillip Watson BSc
School of Sport, Exercise and Health Sciences, Loughborough University, United Kingdom

Chapter 1

The history of sports nutrition: from the early days to the future

Bengt Saltin and Asker Jeukendrup

The Greeks and the Romans

It could be argued that sports nutrition started in paradise when Eve gave the apple to Adam, to make him as strong as God. Nutrition has always intrigued humans. As far back as ancient Greece nutrition has been linked to performance and health. It was Hippocrates (460 BC - ca. 370 BC) who said *"If we could give every individual the right amount of nourishment and exercise, not too little and not too much, we would have found the safest way to health"*. The diet of most Greeks and Romans was predominantly vegetarian and consisted of cereals, fruit, vegetables and legumes, and wine diluted with water. When meat was eaten, the most common source was goat for Greeks and pork for Romans.

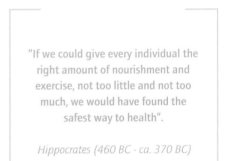

> "If we could give every individual the right amount of nourishment and exercise, not too little and not too much, we would have found the safest way to health".
>
> *Hippocrates (460 BC - ca. 370 BC)*

It is believed that the first documented information about a special diet of a Greek athlete was Charmis of Sparta. He is said to have trained on dried figs. There are other reports of figs being used as sports nutrition. Running was a big part of army training and there were professional runners who were used to send messages sometimes over long distances. The most well known runner was perhaps Pheidipphides, who has been linked to the origin of the marathon. Pheidipphides is said to have run from Athens to Sparta (240km) to ask the Spartans for help when Persians were about to destroy Athens. When the Spartans replied that they were just celebrating an annual ceremony and their laws did not permit them go to Athens to help, Pheidippides had to run back to convey the bad news.

So he ran a total of 480km and he would have used figs as one of his main energy sources. It was estimated that with his 50 kg, he expended 28,000 kcal. (112,000 kJ). He also supposedly ran from Marathon to Athens (40km) which later became the marathon distance at modern Olympic Games). However, whether this run actually took place is still debated.

Olympic Games

According to Galen and other authors, at the end of the third century B.C., athletes believed that drinking herbal teas and eating mushrooms could increase their performance during competition in the ancient Olympic Games (Mottram 1988). There is also a report that states that a meat diet was introduced about the middle of the fifth century by Dromeus of Stymphalos, an ex-long-distance runner. Another account by Diogenes Laertius reports that Eurymenes of Samos consumed a meat diet recommended by his trainer, Pythagoras of Croton. However, by far the best accounts of athletic diet to survive from antiquity are those of Milo of Croton, a wrestler whose feats of strength became legendary and won the wrestling event at five successive Olympics from 532 to 516 B.C. His diet supposedly consisted of 9 kg (20 pounds) of meat, 9 kg (20 pounds) of bread and 8.5 L (18 pints) of wine a day. The validity of these reports from antiquity, however, must be suspect. Although Milo was clearly a large and powerful man, who possessed a prodigious appetite, basic estimations reveal that if he trained on such a volume of food, Milo would have consumed approximately 57,000 kcal (238,500 kJ) per day.

In South America, stimulants like mate tea, coffee and coca were used to increase performance. It has been reported that the Incas chewed coca leaves to cover the distance between Cuzco and Quito, in Ecuador (>1600km).

The first experimental approach

An experimental approach to the field of human muscle energy metabolism had its start in the middle of the 19th century. In 1842 John von Liebig stated that the primary fuel for muscular contraction was protein (Terjung and Horton 1988). However, within two decades this was proven wrong by von Pettenkofer and Voit (1866). Subsequent laboratory experiments focused on whether carbohydrates and fat could be used directly by contracting skeletal muscle. After some initial studies by Chaveux, supporting the view that fat had to be converted to carbohydrates before it could be used by muscle, Zuntz (see Carpenter 1931) claimed that both carbohydrates and fat were oxidized by skeletal muscle, not only at rest but also during exercise. This was confirmed in later studies by Krogh and Lindhard (1920). They also demonstrated that both fuels were used at the same time, in most instances, while protein normally did not play a role as a supplier of energy.

> Initially protein was thought to be the only fuel but soon it was discovered that carbohydrate and fat could be used as fuel and that they were used simultaneously in most situations.

An experimental approach to the field of human muscle energy metabolism had its start in the second part of the 19th century. Before 1900 it was generally thought that protein was the fuel for the muscle. In 1842 John Von Liebig stated that the primary fuel for muscular contraction was protein (see Terjung and Horton 1988). Laboratory experiments with humans were performed to unravel whether carbohydrates and fat could be used directly by contracting skeletal muscle. This laboratory approach gave clear cut answers demonstrating that lipids could be used by human skeletal muscle without first being converted to a sugar. It was found not only that both carbohydrate and fat could be used as a fuel, but in most conditions they are used at the same time. It was also concluded that protein did not play an important role as a fuel (see Terjung and Horton 1988).

At the same time other researchers had a more applied approach searching for the optimal diet for Arctic explorers crossing Ice Caps in the world. The Polar expeditions established that with an energy intake of up to 60-70 % coming from fat, subjects could still maintain a relatively high daily high exercise output. The sledge dogs could, however, perform their heavy task with a diet containing up to 90 % fat.

The importance of carbohydrate feeding

Important observations were also made by Levine and colleagues in the 1920s (Levine et al., 1924). They measured blood glucose concentrations in some of the participants of the 1923 Boston Marathon, which at that time was thought of as an almost impossible, unhealthy and grueling challenge, referred to in some papers as "violent exercise" (Larrabee, 1902). They observed that glucose concentrations markedly declined after the race in most runners. These investigators suggested that low blood glucose levels were a cause of fatigue. To test that hypothesis, they encouraged several participants of the same marathon the following year to consume carbohydrates during the race. This practice, in combination with a high-carbohydrate diet before the race, seemed to prevent hypoglycemia (low blood glucose) and significantly improved running performance (i.e., time to complete the race).

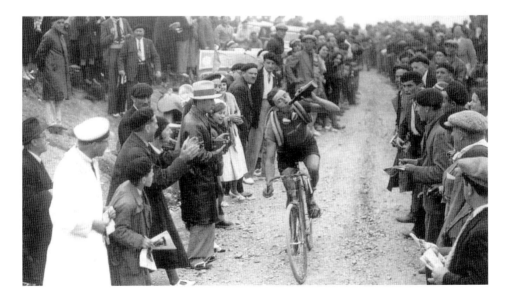

The importance of carbohydrate for improving exercise capacity was further demonstrated by Dill, Edwards, and Talbott (Dill et al., 1932). These investigators let their dogs, Joe and Sally, run without feeding them carbohydrates. The dogs became hypoglycemic and fatigued after 4 to 6 hours. When the test was repeated, with the only difference that the dogs were fed carbohydrates during exercise, the dogs ran for 17 to 23 hours.

Substrate utilization

Since these early days there has been continuous progress in our understanding of the importance of intensity, diet and training status for the substrate choice by skeletal muscle when exercising. Most of the knowledge we have today is derived from studies done in the 1930s. Our understanding of why carbohydrate usage is intensity dependent, why muscle training improves fat utilization and reduces lactate accumulation and why carbohydrate loading elongates time to exhaustion, is still limited.

Methodological improvements in the 1950-60s, such as the use of isotopes and the re-introduction of the biopsy needle (by Jonas Bergström) to take muscle biopsies, brought about new tools for more direct measurements of both substrates used and metabolites produced by muscles. In the 1960s the key role of fatty acids (FA) was recognized as was the storage and usage of muscle glycogen.

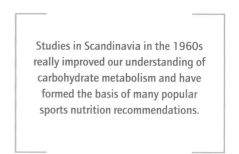

Studies in Scandinavia in the 1960s really improved our understanding of carbohydrate metabolism and have formed the basis of many popular sports nutrition recommendations.

Since the sixties many exercise studies have investigated the relative importance of carbohydrates and fats for energy turnover, which factors limit the oxidation of these substrates and the regulatory mechanisms handling these substrates. There is consensus that fats play a larger role after training but to what extent serum and muscle triglycerides (TG) contribute is intensely debated. There is also debate about what the exact limitation is for the fat utilization during exercise, especially at higher exercise intensities. It has been suggested that the transport of FA into the muscle is the critical step but there is equally strong evidence of a key role for the mitochondrial respiratory capacity. The regulation of the FA uptake by the mitochondria also plays a role.

Although many questions are still unanswered, despite many years of intensive research, it is clear dietary carbohydrates are essential for optimal performance. Equally clear is that a high capacity for lipid oxidation in the active muscles of an endurance athlete is a requirement for optimal endurance performance. In part this is explained by limited glycogen storage capacity but there is probably a lot more to it than that. In the years to come we will learn more about the interactions between the diet and the training of an athlete.

Hydration

In the 80s there were a number of studies showing that dehydration could reduce performance and extreme dehydration could result in heat stroke and adverse health effects. These studies were soon followed up by work to optimize fluid delivery during exercise. Sports drinks appeared on the shelves of sports shops and supermarkets and were marketed toward a growing number of long distance runners and other athletes.

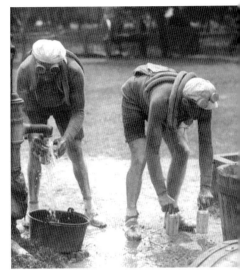

There was clearly a trend towards drinking more and more during endurance events as evidenced by the IAAF (International Athletics Federation) drinking guidelines and regulations for feed stations during marathon races. In 1953 the IAAF handbook for race organizers indicated that feed stations had to be provided only for marathon aces and only at 15 and 30 km. The 2009 guidelines indicate that water should be available at the start and finish of all events, for events up to 10km drinking should be provided every 2-3 km and for longer events refreshment stations have to be provided every 5km. In addition, water should be supplied midway between these refreshment stations. Effectively the total number of drinking opportunities during a marathon may be 17! Over the years the drinking messages got a bit clouded and many runners interpreted the guidelines as a directive to drink as much as possible. However, it is clear that drinking too much water can result in hyponatremia and more recently the drinking advice has stressed that overdrinking can be dangerous (see Chapter 5).

Micronutrients

Micronutrients have received some attention too. Since their discovery, vitamins have been more or less synonymous with good health because it was clear that a lack of these essential nutrients resulted in illness. Since the 40s and 50s it became common practice for sports people to supplement with vitamins in order to perform better. However, research consistently indicated that as long as there were no deficiencies, vitamin intakes over and above the daily recommended amounts did not enhance performance. Nevertheless, the use of vitamins and minerals, and antioxidants in particular, is still very popular. More recently, however, studies pointed out that large amounts of antioxidants could actually prevent (or at least reduce) normal training adaptations. It has also become clear that large doses of certain vitamins and minerals can have detrimental health effects.

The final note is a tribute to the early researchers in the field and to their accomplishments. Not only is reading their work enjoyable, we have also gained tremendous knowledge from their work. They contributed greatly to both to the applied aspects as well as our more fundamental understanding of possible limiting factors in endurance sports.

Chapter 2

What is the optimal composition of an athlete's diet?

Liz Broad and Greg Cox

The optimal composition

There is much debate about what athletes should eat and what the optimal composition of an athlete's diet is. How much carbohydrate should it contain, how much fat and how much protein? Are vitamin and mineral requirements increased? The fact is that there is no one optimal diet for all athletes. The optimal composition of an athlete's diet will depend on the sport the athlete engages in, the amount and type of training the athlete undertakes, and whether the athlete needs to manipulate their body weight or body composition. In brief, athletes need an individualized nutrition plan that is based on sound scientific principles and that is easily incorporated into their daily routine. This interface – the conversion of science into food – is where a skilled sports nutrition professional can apply their expertise. However, there are a few simple guidelines.

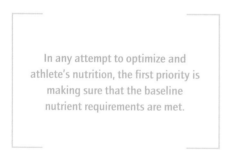

In any attempt to optimize and athlete's nutrition, the first priority is making sure that the baseline nutrient requirements are met.

Where to start?

The first priority is to consider baseline nutrient requirements. Fortunately these fall in line with recommendations for the general population in terms of most micronutrient (vitamins, minerals, fiber) needs and general trends in terms of the balance of macronutrients (carbohydrate, fat, protein and alcohol). This generally requires eating a variety of foods from all basic food groups, and creating a structure whereby food is distributed consistently throughout the day rather than at one or two time points. Once achieved, specific timing, quantities and food choices can be tailored to meet sport-specific requirements of the athlete.

One starting point could be to determine daily protein needs. Over the years, there has been a great deal of debate regarding the optimal protein intake of athletes. It is important to distinguish between requirements to maintain good health and the protein needs to optimize muscle growth and other adaptations to training.

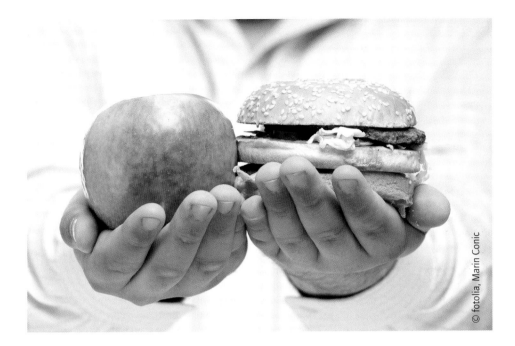

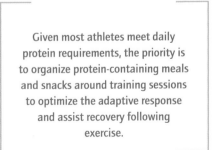

© fotolia, Marin Conic

Protein: the building blocks

The general recommendation for protein intake is in the range of 1.2-1.7 g·kg BM^{-1}·d^{-1}, regardless of type of exercise. (See Chapters 7, 9 and 11 in this book.) Dietary intake surveys of athletes frequently report that protein requirements are more than adequately met by the vast majority of athletes. However, some athletes have become overzealous with their focus on consuming protein, neglecting the importance of balance and fueling exercise or reducing carbohydrate intake in an attempt to reduce body fat levels. Given most athletes meet daily protein requirements because their energy intake increases to match training loads, the priority is to organize protein-containing meals and snacks around training sessions to optimize the adaptive response and assist recovery following exercise. For example, consuming a snack that provides 10-20g of protein immediately after resistance training for a rugby union player requires education and forward planning. Once their protein intake is planned to support training, the remainder can be distributed into the other meals and snacks to ensure a range of different food sources are used to meet essential nutrient requirements such as calcium (i.e. 3-4 servings of dairy), iron and zinc.

> Given most athletes meet daily protein requirements, the priority is to organize protein-containing meals and snacks around training sessions to optimize the adaptive response and assist recovery following exercise.

Carbohydrate: the preferred energy source

The other important macronutrient is carbohydrate, the predominant fuel source in moderate to high intensity exercise. It is now widely acknowledged that general recommendations for daily carbohydrate intake should be expressed as grams of carbohydrate per kilogram of the athlete's body mass rather than a percentage of total dietary energy (Burke et al. 2001). Suggested carbohydrate intake guidelines for athletes based on daily exercise patterns and expressed relative to an athlete's body weight have been recently developed (see Table 1). Interpretation of these guidelines into an athlete's dietary plan should consider the athlete's overall daily energy requirements, specific training volume and intensity, and requirements for growth and development (for children and adolescent athletes). Without an inherent knowledge of a sport, these guidelines can be easily misinterpreted. For example, it is not uncommon for a gymnast to train for 6-7 hours per day, over two training sessions. If you consider the training sessions duration alone, this would place their carbohydrate requirements at 10-12+$g \cdot kg^{-1}$ BM$\cdot d^{-1}$ according to current recommendations. In reality when the absolute amount of 'activity' is calculated within total training hours, the estimated amount of energy expended is quite small and has been estimated at 0.066 kcal$\cdot min^{-1} \cdot kg^{-1}$. The net result of true exercise energy expenditure in the sessions for an average 50 kg gymnast adds only 1200 kcal (5000 kJ) to their daily energy requirements. However, if the athlete consumed the amount based on training time alone of 10 g carbohydrate$\cdot kg$ BM$^{-1} \cdot d^{-1}$ (equivalent to over 8000kJ), this would well exceed the energy expenditure of exercise, and thus highlights the need to 'know your sport'. Although we have no definitive assessment of carbohydrate usage during gymnastics training, it is likely daily requirements are within 5-6 $g \cdot kg$ BM$^{-1} \cdot d^{-1}$. As an alternate example, a 110 kg rugby union prop who trains twice a day in both strength and field sessions, incorporating high intensity bouts of exercise, would theoretically have carbohydrate requirements of 7-12 $g \cdot kg$ BM$^{-1} \cdot d^{-1}$, or >770 g carbohydrate$\cdot day$. Functionally, it is very difficult for these players to find the time and the capacity to eat that amount of carbohydrate. In reality, these players appear to train and recover well when carbohydrate intake is closer to 5-6 $g \cdot kg$ BM$^{-1} \cdot d^{-1}$.

> Carbohydrate intake guidelines for athletes based on daily exercise patterns and expressed relative to an athlete's body weight have been developed. However, these guidelines have to be interpreted with caution and an inherent knowledge of a sport and its energy requirements is required.

Carbohydrate when recovery times are short

When there is little time to recover (2-8h) it is important to make sure muscle fuel (glycogen) stores are restored as quickly as possible. To promote optimal glycogen recovery it is recommended to ingest 1 g of carbohydrate$\cdot kg$ BM as soon as practical following the session.

This can be achieved by incorporating additional recovery snacks or, alternatively for athletes with a low energy budget, rescheduling the timing of the next meal (see Chapter 7). This can then be followed up with a similar amount in the subsequent 2h period if restoration of glycogen stores is the priority, as is the case following hard or prolonged workouts when training multiple times throughout the day. Consider whether you require carbohydrate *during* or *before* training, based on the goals of the training session itself and the relative importance of maintaining a strong work output throughout the entire session versus using the session to promote the metabolic and physiological adaptations to training. Once you have allocated appropriate carbohydrate to this, then as with protein, distribute the remainder of your requirements throughout the other meals and snacks for the day, using a range of different foods. In this instance, make sure this includes fruit and vegetables for their antioxidant content rather than making the carbohydrate predominantly cereal-based, and don't leave it all to the last meal of the day. For those with very high energy needs, lower fiber options and liquid options (juice, cordial, flavored milks, etc.) are useful inclusions as otherwise the diet becomes too bulky.

Fat intake modified to meet remaining goals

Every athlete has an energy 'budget' which reflects their energy expenditure as well as body composition goals. Targets set for body fat/mass loss should be moderate (250-500 kcal or 1200-2000 kJ less than estimated daily energy expenditure), and similarly increased for muscle mass gain. The first priority is to meet daily protein and carbohydrate requirements to support training and facilitate recovery within this energy budget (see Chapter 20). This may mean reducing dietary fat intake (due to its high energy content) for athletes with a low energy budget (i.e. those trying to decrease body fat stores). Alternatively, there may be room to increase intakes of all 3 macronutrients to achieve energy demands. Most foods contain several different types of fats as evidenced on food labels. It's important when choosing dietary fats, and fat-containing foods, that consideration be given to essential fat–soluble vitamins and essential fatty acids, as well as understanding the role of different dietary fats in lifestyle related disease and inflammatory processes. Good choices include consuming nutritious food sources of fats (such as avocadoes, oily fish, and nuts) and healthier sources of fats (olive oil, polyunsaturated oils, and canola oil).

The practicalities of developing a nutrition plan

For athletes who undertake routine daily training with little variation from one day to the next, it's common practice among sports nutrition professionals to develop an individualized food and fluid intake plan based on an estimated average daily energy expenditure. For instance, divers typically undertake 2 hours of dry-land training in the morning, and 3 hours of afternoon diving practice. This daily routine is followed 5-6 days a week, with only minor adjustments in daily workloads. In this case differences in daily energy expenditure are minimal and are easily accommodated with a generic daily food and fluid plan that may only change in terms of food selection and variety.

An alternate approach is to develop a meal plan which can cater to athletes that have large daily fluctuations in training. For instance, a triathlete may undertake 6-8 hours of training including a mix of sustained aerobic activity and repeated bouts of high intensity efforts on high training days; and an easy 30-40 minute jog on their weekly rest day. In developing a meal plan for athletes with large daily fluctuations in energy expenditure, it's important to ensure the daily meal plan can be easily manipulated by the athlete to compensate for changes in exercise patterns. Additional energy (namely in the form of carbohydrate) can be included before, during or after training to support daily exercise performance and recovery between exercise sessions. Of interest, Saris and colleagues (1989) found that male cyclists contesting the Tour de France modified their daily carbohydrate and energy intakes to reflect daily energy expenditure when supported by a professional team. Cyclists in this study consumed 94 grams of carbohydrate each hour while racing which accounted for almost half (49%) of their total daily energy intake. By comparison, Burke et al. (2003) found that male team and endurance athletes reported consuming only 3-5% of their total energy intake during training. The striking disparity between these two studies is likely to be a reflection of the organized support offered to elite cyclists by their professional team and the emphasis on maintaining 'best' performance from one day to the next throughout the course of the event. The take home message for athletes and coaches is to be organized and strategic when including additional foods and fluid to support the demands of training. This can only be achieved with forward planning and access to suitable foods and fluids.

> An individualized food and fluid intake plan is usually based on an estimated average daily energy expenditure.

Finally, athletes are faced with the added challenge of eating socially among family, friends, team mates and colleagues (for non-professional athletes). As clinical as sports nutrition guidelines may appear, athletes do not eat solely to support exercise performance and promote recovery between exercise sessions. Athletes must strike a balance to ensure they optimize their intake to support training and competition performances, while maintaining a flexible approach and attitude towards food to engage in social activities away from sport. Athletes and coaches are advised to seek advice from a sports nutrition professional who can help you achieve your goals.

Table 1: Guidelines for Carbohydrate (CHO) intakes in everyday training

Activity	CHO Intake (g·kg BM^{-1}·d^{-1})
Immediate recovery after exercise (0-4 h)	1.0-1.2 g·kg BM^{-1}·h^{-1}
Minimal physical activity	2-3
Light physical activity (3-5 h·wk)	4-5
Daily recovery: moderate duration and intensity training (10 h·wk)	5-7
Daily recovery: moderate to heavy endurance training (20+ h·wk)	7-12
Daily recovery: extreme exercise program (4-6+ h·day)	10-12+

Chapter 3

The optimal pre-competition meal

Asker Jeukendrup

Even textbooks are sometimes confusing when it comes to pre-exercise meals. Some books will tell you to avoid carbohydrate (CHO) in the hour before exercise and some will tell you that you need it to improve performance. The last big meal is often planned 3-4 hours before a race but what should you eat and how much?

CHO loading in the days prior to exercise

The classic studies from Scandinavia in the late sixties that demonstrated the importance of muscle glycogen resulted in the development of a glycogen super compensation diet (see Chapter 1). Glycogen depletion in combination with a high carbohydrate intake resulted in a marked increase (super compensation) in muscle glycogen and enhanced subsequent endurance exercise performance. The proposed protocol to achieve these very high glycogen stores was pretty extreme and involved an exhausting exercise bout, no training at all for 6 days, a diet that consisted almost entirely of fat (3d), followed by a diet consisting almost entirely of carbohydrate (3d) (see Table 1). More recently, a less extreme diet-exercise regimen was almost equally effective in elevating pre-exercise muscle glycogen to these levels. With this moderate glycogen loading protocol it has also been shown that trained athletes can increase their muscle glycogen to very high levels in as little as one day by ingesting 10 g $CHO \cdot kg^{-1}$ body mass and remaining inactive. Muscle glycogen did not increase further during another 2 days of rest and high CHO intake. There is also evidence that well-trained athletes can maintain, or even increase, their muscle glycogen stores to very high levels in less than 24 h while training (67% VO_2 peak) 2 h per day and consuming 10-12.5 g $CHO \cdot kg^{-1}$ body mass per day. It has even been suggested that trained athletes can greatly increase

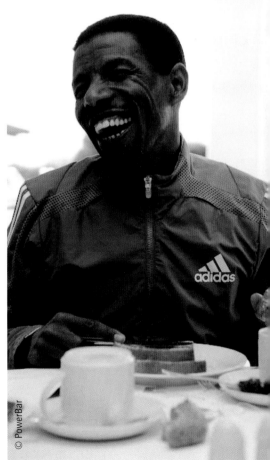
© PowerBar

their muscle glycogen stores in <24 h by performing only 3 min of supramaximal exercise and then consuming a high CHO diet. This protocol potentially represents an improvement over previous regimens that have been extensively tested under laboratory and/or field conditions and further study is warranted.

> Complicated strategies to glycogen load and 'super compensate' are not essential to achieve very high muscle glycogen concentrations prior to competition.

Despite a greater reliance on muscle glycogen when pre-exercise levels are elevated, increased dietary CHO in the 1-7 days prior to exercise is generally associated with enhanced performance when exercise duration exceeds 90 minutes. This is most likely due to a delay in the point at which muscle glycogen availability is limiting for optimal exercise performance. The largest effects are observed during exercise trials to exhaustion (often referred to as endurance "capacity") and are smaller in magnitude during tests of endurance "performance" that are not open-ended such as total work output in a given time or time taken to complete a certain distance or amount of work. During prolonged, strenuous exercise, rates of carbohydrate oxidation can be as high as 3-4 g$\cdot$min^{-1}, derived primarily from muscle glycogen.

CHO loading does not appear to further increase exercise performance when CHO availability is maintained high with a pre-exercise CHO meal and CHO ingestion during exercise.

Team sports and sprints

In shorter, more intense exercise bouts the benefits of glycogen loading are not apparent, probably because muscle glycogen availability is not a limiting factor in the non-CHO loaded trial in this type of exercise.

During single bouts of high intensity exercise, the effects of CHO loading are somewhat equivocal. Some studies have observed enhanced performance with elevated muscle glycogen levels following increased dietary CHO intake, while other investigators have observed no benefit of elevated pre-exercise muscle glycogen. In some of the studies the differences in performance were most obvious at the extremes of diet and may have been due as much to deleterious acid-base disturbances following consumption of a high fat-protein diet as to increased muscle glycogen availability following the high CHO diet.

With repeated bouts of high intensity exercise, increased muscle glycogen availability is associated with enhanced intermittent exercise performance (Balsom et al. 1999). Furthermore, increasing dietary CHO intake from 300 g$\cdot$day^{-1} to 600 g$\cdot$day^{-1} for two days prior to exercise improved long-term, intermittent exercise performance (Bangsbo et al. 1992), while ingestion of 10g CHO$\cdot$kg^{-1} body mass improved intermittent running capacity during 22 h of recovery when compared with an isoenergetic diet without additional CHO (Nicholas et al. 1997).

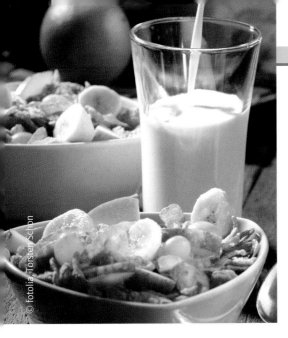

It has been suggested that females may have a reduced ability to increase muscle glycogen levels during a period of dietary CHO loading but more recently it has been shown that with adequate energy and CHO intake, female athletes benefit from CHO loading as much as male athletes (see Chapter 15).

In conclusion CHO loading the days before competition is relevant for some but not all sports. The protocol employed to achieve this may depend on practicalities such a training and available time.

Carbohydrate 3-4 hours prior to exercise

Ingestion of a CHO-rich meal (containing 140 - 330 g CHO) 3-4 h prior to exercise has been shown increase muscle glycogen levels and enhance exercise performance. An increase in pre-exercise muscle glycogen is one explanation for the enhanced performance. Alternatively, because liver glycogen levels are substantially reduced after an overnight fast, ingestion of CHO may increase these reserves and contribute, together with any ongoing absorption of the ingested CHO, to the maintenance of blood glucose levels and improved performance during subsequent exercise (Casey et al. 2000).

Despite plasma glucose and insulin levels returning to basal levels, ingestion of CHO in the hours prior to exercise often results in a transient fall in glucose with the onset of exercise, increased CHO oxidation and a blunting of fatty acid (FA) mobilization. These metabolic perturbations can

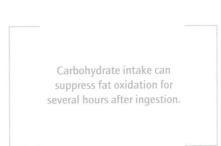

Carbohydrate intake can suppress fat oxidation for several hours after ingestion.

persist for up to 6 h following CHO ingestion (Montain et al. 1991), but are not detrimental to exercise performance. Ann increased CHO availability apparently compensates for the greater CHO utilization. No differences in exercise performance have been observed following ingestion of meals that produced marked differences in plasma glucose and insulin levels (Wee et al. 1999). The effects of a high CHO meal 3-4 h prior to exercise on subsequent performance may be equivalent to those observed with CHO ingestion during exercise (Chryssanthopoulos et al., 1994), although this is not always the case (Wright et al. 1991) and there may be some important metabolic differences. The combination of a pre-exercise CHO meal and CHO ingestion during exercise may further enhance exercise performance (Wright et al. 1991). From a practical perspective, if access to CHO during exercise is limited or nonexistent, ingestion of 200-300 g CHO 3-4 h prior to exercise may be an effective strategy for enhancing CHO availability during the subsequent exercise period. Furthermore, ingestion of CHO may be effective in enhancing subsequent exercise performance when the recovery period is relatively short (4 h, (Fallowfield et al. 1995)).

> If access to CHO during exercise is limited or nonexistent, ingestion of 200-300 g CHO 3-4 h prior to exercise may be an effective strategy for enhancing CHO availability during the subsequent exercise period.

What to eat in the hour before a race?

As mentioned above, even textbooks are sometimes confusing when it comes to pre-exercise meals. Some books will tell you to avoid carbohydrate in the hour before exercise and some will tell you that you need it to improve performance. The reason for these different views stems from a couple of early studies. In these studies in the 70s, it was observed that eating carbohydrate in the hour before exercise resulted in high blood glucose and insulin concentrations at the start of exercise. Then, as exercise started there was a rapid drop of the blood glucose concentrations because of a combined effect of hyperinsulinemia and exercise on glucose uptake. Blood glucose concentrations dropped so much that hypoglycemia occurred. This is often called rebound hypoglycemia or reactive hypoglycemia and is associated with symptoms of weakness, nausea and dizziness and is thought to have a negative impact on performance. In fact one of the early studies reported that performance was reduced when carbohydrate was ingested before exercise compared with placebo (water) ingestion.

Since then, numerous studies have been performed. Some of these studies investigated carbohydrates that do not result in a large insulin response (low glycemic index carbohydrates) such as fructose. These studies (over a hundred from different research groups all over the world) showed either no effect of carbohydrate feeding on performance or a positive effect. All these different studies used different types of carbohydrates, different modes and intensities of exercise, different subjects (some trained, some untrained). This made it difficult to compare the results and very difficult to find out exactly what caused the different effects. However, more recently we performed a series of studies in which we examined the effects of pre-exercise carbohydrate feedings very systematically (Achten et al. 2003; Jentjens et al. 2002a; Jentjens et al. 2002b, 2003; Moseley et al. 2003). All studies had a similar design and we only changed one variable at a time. The overall conclusion of these studies was that there was no effect on performance even though in some cases hypoglycemia did develop. There was no relation at all between the blood

> There is *no* reason *not* to consume carbohydrate before exercise as there do not seem to be any detrimental effects on performance. Individuals prone to developing reactive hypoglycemia can find solutions to avoid it.

glucose concentrations and performance. Hypoglycemia was more prevalent when smaller amounts of carbohydrate were ingested (25g) compared with larger amounts (75g or 200g) 45 min before. Hypoglycemia is less prevalent when it is ingested just (15 min) before exercise compared with 45 and 75 min before. Low glycemic index carbohydrates do not cause hypoglycemia.

An interesting finding was that some individuals developed hypoglycemia in all conditions whereas other did not develop hypoglycemia regardless of the condition, confirming anecdotal evidence that some individuals are more likely to develop hypoglycemia than others. Somewhat surprisingly, this was not linked to insulin sensitivity of the individual. A list of ways to avoid hypoglycemia can be found in Table 2.

In practical terms this means that there is *no* reason *not* to consume carbohydrate before exercise as there do not seem to be any detrimental effects on performance. Individuals prone of developing reactive hypoglycemia can find solutions to avoid it. These solutions could include choosing low glycemic index carbohydrates, ingesting carbohydrate just before exercise or during a warm up or avoiding carbohydrate in the 90 min before.

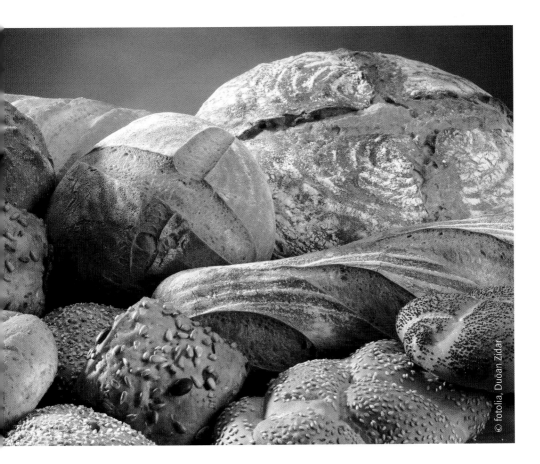

© fotolia, Dušan Zidar

Table 1: Glycogen loading strategies

Glycogen loading protocol	Description	Muscle glycogen (mmol·kg ww)
Classical glycogen loading protocol	Glycogen depletion followed by 3 days very high fat (no carbohydrate) diet, and 3 days high carbohydrate (no fat diet)	800-1000
Moderate glycogen loading protocol	As training is reduced towards and event the carbohydrate intake increases from 50-60% to 80%.	700-800
High intensity exercise and very high CHO diet	3 min of supramaximal exercise followed by a high CHO diet can increase glycogen stores to very high levels within 24h	700-800
High carbohydrate, very low fat diet while continuing training	Subjects train 2h per day at 65% VO_2max and consume a diet with 10-12·5 g $CHO \cdot kg^{-1}$ body mass per day. This means that fat content in the diet is extremely low (and may affect intramuscular fat stores)	800-1000
A typical diet and minimal exercise	A typical diet with 5 g $CHO \cdot kg^{-1}$ body mass per day and minimal exercise (1 h per day)	400-500

Table 2: Ways to reduce the risk of rebound hypoglycemia

Avoid CHO in the hour before exercise
Eat/drink CHO in the last 5 min before the start
Eat/drink CHO during the warm-up
Choose moderate to low glycemic index CHO sources
If you ingest CHO in the hour before, ingest (larger) amounts >60g
Don't start too fast (if this is possible)
Once exercise has started, keep ingesting CHO

Chapter 4

Carbohydrate intake during exercise: when, what and how much?

Asker Jeukendrup

The benefits of carbohydrate ingestion during endurance exercise are well described and known since the 80s. Since then, research has focused on optimizing the supply of carbohydrates and answering practical questions like, When does the carbohydrate have to be ingested? What types of carbohydrates and how much needs to be ingested?

Carbohydrates during prolonged exercise work

The fact that carbohydrate intake during prolonged exercise can enhance exercise performance is known since the 80s. Even in the 1920s suggestions were made that taking sugar during a marathon could improve performance (see Chapter 1). The ingested carbohydrate simply provides an extra fuel, thereby sparing your body carbohydrate stores. During exercise blood glucose concentrations are maintained with carbohydrate feeding as they would drop to low levels within 2-3 hours if no carbohydrate was ingested. The carbohydrate intake also helps to maintain high rates of carbohydrate utilization by the muscle which ultimately helps maintain power.

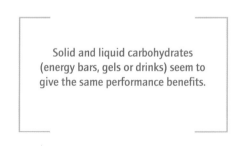

Solid and liquid carbohydrates (energy bars, gels or drinks) seem to give the same performance benefits.

It has therefore been advised to take carbohydrate on board in all races that last 2 hours or longer. Carbohydrate may also help performance in team sports especially those lasting >60 min (Currell et al. 2009) and during exercise of approximately 1 hour duration (Carter et al. 2004) but the mechanisms may be very different. (See Chapter 18 for more detail.)

Studies have shown that the form in which these carbohydrates are ingested is not really important. Solid and liquid carbohydrates (energy bars, gels or drinks) seem to give the same performance benefits. When racing it is important to stay hydrated, especially in hot conditions. The ingestion of solid food will slow down gastric emptying and may consequently slow down the delivery of fluids. On the other hand, solid foods will give you a more satisfying feeling in your stomach, which can be important in longer races.

The type and amount of carbohydrate matter

The type of carbohydrate may have a major impact on the efficacy (Jeukendrup 2000, 2004, 2005). The muscle can use some carbohydrates at higher rates than others and this is most likely related to the different absorption rates of carbohydrates. Glucose, sucrose (table sugar) and maltodextrins (a chain of 10-16 glucose molecules), common ingredients in sports drinks, are all rapidly utilized (see Table 1). Fructose, galactose, and some starches are utilized at much lower rates. Here we will refer to these as the slow carbohydrates.

> The most sensible advice would be to ingest between 20 and 70 grams of carbohydrate per hour. In some situations it may be better to take up to 90 grams per hour but this should be from multiple transportable carbohydrates (i.e. glucose and fructose).

The amount of carbohydrate you ingest has an impact too. Early studies have shown that the ingestion of as little as 20 grams per hour can result in performance improvements. More recent studies seem to suggest that taking more carbohydrate from your drinks can result in a further performance improvement (Currell et al. 2008). However, it has also been shown that the maximum rate at which carbohydrate can be used from a drink is about 60 grams per hour. Even when very large amounts of carbohydrate are ingested (120 to 180 grams per hour), this does not result in higher oxidation rates and the carbohydrate simply accumulates in the stomach and intestine which is likely to cause gastrointestinal discomfort.

Ingesting much more than 60 grams per hour would have no further effect. The most sensible advice would therefore be to ingest at least 20 and up to about 70 grams of carbohydrate per hour. Ways to increase this to >90 grams per hour will be discussed later. In practical terms, since most sports drinks contain mainly one type of carbohydrate, it would be safe to work with intakes up to 70 grams per hour.

Table 1: Ingested carbohydrates are oxidiused at different rates

Low oxidation rates	High oxidation rates	Very high oxidation rates
Galactose	Glucose	Glucose:fructose*
Fructose	Sucrose	Maltodextrin:fructose*
Trehalose	Maltose	Glucose: sucrose:fructose*
Isomaltulose	Maltodextrin	
Amylose starch	Amylopectin starch	

Glucose and maltodextrins should be supplied in amounts that saturate the intestinal transporters (60 g•h). Fructose should be supplied in sufficient quantities (2:1 glucose:fructose ratio or more).

Carbohydrate in practice

So how can the above information be used in a long distance race? This depends, of course, on your sport and the opportunities you will have to take carbohydrate sources with you or be supplied with drinks during the race. In some races (cycling, for example) it is possible to take a reasonable amount of energy from the start. In other races (marathon) it is difficult to take much and you will have to rely more on what will be provided. You can prepare your own drink from scratch or you can buy a commercially available sports drink. In team sports carbohydrate intake is usually restricted to before the game and at half time. Plan your nutrition so that your carbohydrate intake is approximately 60-70 grams every hour. You can achieve this intake by selecting bars, gels and drinks. For example, a gel will typically contain 25 grams of carbohydrate, a bar may contain 20-30 grams and half a liter of a sports drink will provide approximately 30-40 grams. By combining these different carbohydrate sources you can get an intake of 60-70 grams per hour. It is important to drink water with the bars and gels so that absorption is accelerated and hydration is maintained. How much you need to drink depends on fluid loss (sweat rate). Guidelines for fluid delivery will be discussed in later chapters. Depending on the situation, it may be more convenient to carry drinks, gels or bars. During a marathon carrying drinks is not practical. Carrying gels would be easier and water is supplied by the organizers.

> The desired carbohydrate intake can be achieved by consuming carbohydrate drinks, gels and bars or a combination thereof.

Recent studies suggest that carbohydrate delivery can be boosted by taking carbohydrates in certain combinations. This will also be discussed in Chapter 12 and 25.

The ideal sports drink

Based on the information so far, your ideal sports drink should fulfill a number of criteria:

- It should taste good. If you don't like the drink you will drink less which has consequences in terms of both fluid and carbohydrate intake.
- It should not cause any gastrointestinal discomfort. Some drinks cause stomach problems and this is highly individual. You may be able to tolerate drink A but not drink B, whereas another person may tolerate drink B but not A.)
- The drink should provide 60-70 grams of carbohydrate per hour in a concentration not higher than about 8% (which is 80 grams per liter). (For long distance events this may be increased to 90 grams per hour with the ingestion of multiple transportable carbohydrates (see below).)
- The drink should contain sodium (to help fluid absorption).
- The drink should not contain too many other salts. (Some drinks are overloaded.)

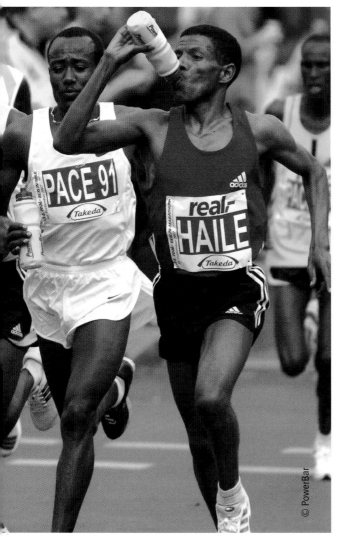

© PowerBar

It cannot be emphasized enough that you should not experiment with new drinks in a race or competition. Sometimes drinks simply cannot be tolerated very well and it would be a shame to find out in such a situation! So be prepared, find out what drinks are available in races and train regularly with these drinks! It is also important to note that the gut is extremely adaptable and can get used to new drinks and larger amounts of carbohydrate. It is well known that runners usually do not drink a lot during a marathon. It is often said that the drinks cannot be tolerated. One of the main reasons they cannot be tolerated is the fact that they have not used these drinks in training. These drinks will be tolerated much better if used on a regular basis during training and performance may improve!

What's new?

Recent scientific developments have focused on improving the carbohydrate delivery from drinks and certain combinations of different types of carbohydrate. For example, glucose and fructose have been shown to improve the delivery of carbohydrates by up to 75% compared to what was previously thought to be "maximal carbohydrate delivery"! The reason why oxidation of carbohydrate from a drink is limited, to about 60 grams per hour, is that the transporters in the intestine become saturated and simply work at full capacity to supply 60 grams of carbohydrate per hour (see Figure 1). In order to increase the total amount of carbohydrate that is absorbed into the body a second carbohydrate can be used that makes use of a different intestinal transporter. Glucose and fructose use different transporters and when they are used in combination absorption and oxidation of ingested carbohydrate can be increased significantly (Figure 1). This may have several advantages: 1) more energy delivery; 2) larger amounts of the ingested carbohydrate are absorbed leaving less in the intestine which can potentially reduce the risk of gastro-intestinal problems; 3) with more carbohydrates being transported water flows in the same direction which improves fluid delivery as well.

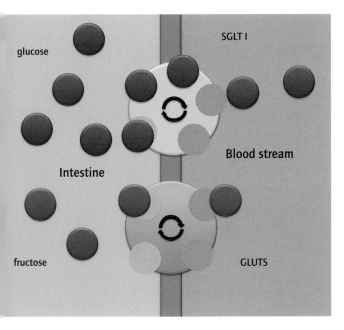

Figure 1: Absorption of carbohydrates in the intestine. Glucose and fructose use different transporters (SGLT1 and GLUT5, respectively). When the glucose transporter SGLT1 becomes saturated, total carbohydrate absorption (and this delivery to the working muscle) can only be increased by using an additional carbohydrate (fructose) that uses a different transporter (GLUT5).

Studies are also emerging which show that high oxidation rates of the carbohydrate can be beneficial to performance in some situations (Table 2). In one study it was demonstrated that performance was enhanced by 8% with a glucose:fructose mixture compared with glucose only (Currell et al. 2008). In this study subjects exercised for 2 hours followed by the equivalent of a 40km time trial. Glucose improved performance by 9%. In contrast, the glucose:fructose improved performance by an additional 8%! It must be noted however that such effects will require the ingestion of fairly large amounts of carbohydrate, which, in itself, could be linked to gastro-intestinal problems. Combinations of carbohydrates (for example, glucose and fructose) ingested at high rates seem to minimize the negative side effects and optimize carbohydrate delivery. A practical example of such carbohydrate intake will be discussed in Chapter 25.

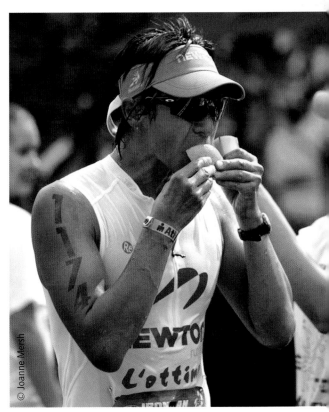

© Joanne Mersh

Table 2: Carbohydrate intake advice for different endurance events

EVENT	CHOICE OF CARBOHYDRATE			
	Energy expenditure	Carbohydrate required for optimal performance and minimizing negative energy balance	Recommended intake	Carbohydrate type
Exercise of <45 min duration	>18 kcal·min^{-1}	No CHO required	*	*
Exercise of 1 h duration	14-18 kcal·min^{-1}	Very small amounts of CHO	*	*
Exercise >2 h Low to moderate intensity	5-7 kcal·min^{-1}	Small amounts of CHO	Up to 30 g·h^{-1}	Can be achieved with most forms of CHO
Exercise >2 h Moderate to high intensity	7-10 kcal·min^{-1}	Moderate amounts of CHO	Up to 60 g·h^{-1}	Can be achieved with CHOs that are rapidly oxidized
Ironman, Tour de France stage races	10-14 kcal·min^{-1}	Large amounts of CHO	Up to 90 g·h^{-1}	Can only be achieved by intakes of multiple transportable CHO

Strategies to take carbohydrate on board

When Carbohydrate ingestion can enhance performance during exercise of 45 min or longer. So in competition or when the quality of a training session is important, consuming some form of carbohydrate will help.

What The type of carbohydrate has considerable impact on the speed of energy delivery. Some carbohydrates are oxidized at higher rates than others. However, a combination of maltodextrins and fructose, glucose and fructose, or glucose, sucrose and fructose seems to result in the highest oxidation rates.

How the carbohydrate is ingested, and in what form, seems to be less important for the delivery of carbohydrate than for fluid delivery. Highly concentrated carbohydrate solutions can impair fluid delivery. It is generally recommended to ingest a certain volume at the start to prime the stomach and to keep topping this up with smaller boluses at regular intervals.

How much Your requirements depend on a number of factors: 1) the type of exercise (intensity and duration) (see Table 1); 2) the type of carbohydrate (or combination of carbohydrates); 3) your individual tolerance which (when determined in the course of and by training (and competition)) will help you find out what will work to your advantage.

Chapter 5

Hydration: what is new?

Asker Jeukendrup

The topic of hydration has received considerable attention in the last few years and there has been debate about the recommendations that should be given to athletes. Reports of overdrinking and resulting hyponatremia have raised questions about current fluid intake practices and the guidelines have been challenged. In addition to hydration, it is also important to provide fuel during prolonged exercise. Therefore, we are seeking the best ways to provide fuel and fluid at the same time.

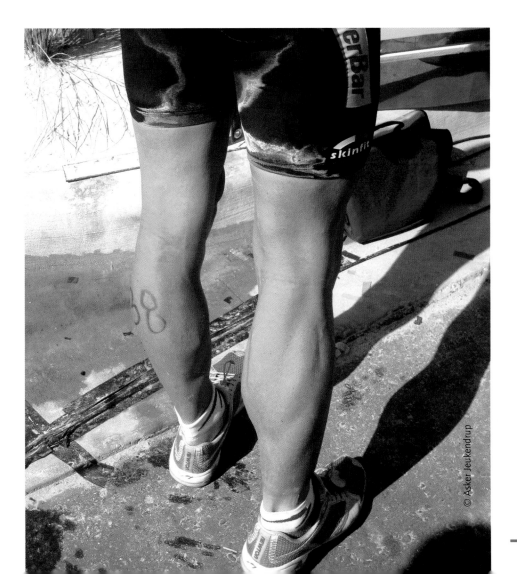

© Asker Jeukendrup

Dehydration impairs performance: the evidence

Fatigue toward the end of a prolonged sporting event is typically multifaceted and the underlying mechanisms are complex. Fatigue may be influenced by dehydration as well as by fuel substrate depletion. It has been demonstrated that exercise performance can be impaired when an individual is dehydrated by as little as 2% of body weight. Losses in excess of 5% of body weight can decrease the capacity for work by about 30%. Even high intensity exercise may be affected by dehydration. In cool laboratory conditions, maximal aerobic power decreases by about 5% when persons experience fluid losses equivalent to 3% of body mass or more. In hot conditions, similar water deficits can cause a larger decrease in VO_2max. Endurance capacity is impaired much more in hot environments than in cool conditions, which suggests that impaired thermoregulation is an important causal factor in the reduced exercise performance associated with a body-water deficit. Severe dehydration also poses a health risk given that it increases the risk of cramps, heat exhaustion, and (life-threatening) heat stroke.

Studies have also shown that fluid ingestion during exercise helps to restore plasma volume to near pre-exercise levels and prevents adverse effects of dehydration on muscle strength, endurance, and coordination. It was argued that relying on feeling thirsty as the signal to drink is unreliable because a considerable degree of dehydration (certainly sufficient to impair athletic performance) can occur before the desire for fluid intake is evident. This is where the debate is heating up (Sawka et al. 2007b).

The debate

Although there is a significant body of evidence that dehydration can impair exercise performance, Professor Noakes has warned, that the extrapolation of these mostly laboratory studies to a real life situation can be problematic (Noakes 2007a, 2007b). Instead of advising to drink to avoid dehydration, Noakes advocates drinking according to thirst (Noakes 2007a, 2007b).

Dr. Noakes argues that "thirst" and not "dehydration" is the factor that determines performance. Thirst is part of a complex mechanism, regulated centrally in the brain, the goal of which is to ensure that athletes do not damage their health by continuing to exercise while drinking too little during exercise.

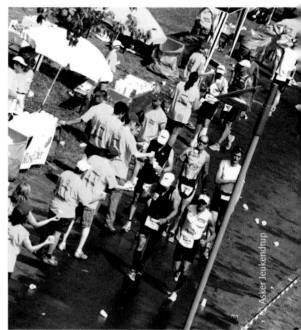

© Asker Jeukendrup

Thirst is driven by the level of "dehydration" which is detected by the brain as a change in plasma osmolality (thickness of the plasma). Osmolality will be one of the key homeostatic variables that a complex system will actively regulate during exercise. According to Noakes' interpretation, "dehydration" is not the direct "cause" of an impaired exercise performance. Rather, exercise performance is modified (impaired) under certain stressful conditions in order to ensure that the osmolality of the brain remains within the homeostatic range. Dr. Noakes also argues that the common advice of drinking before you get thirsty and drinking to prevent dehydration may sometimes result in overdrinking with hyponatremia as a possible consequence. Finally he makes the point that dehydration may sometimes be beneficial to performance as the fastest runners in a marathon are the ones who are dehydrated the most.

Thirst is a basic physiological instinct that the body uses to maintain normal thickness of body fluids. Part of Dr. Noakes' reasoning is that humans evolved the thirst mechanism over millennia and it is the only system used by all other creatures on this earth. Why should it not also be ideal for humans?

The guidelines

Until the early 1970s, the guidelines for fluid ingestion during exercise were not to drink. In the years following years studies demonstrated that performance was reduced by dehydration and was enhanced when fluid was ingested (compared with no fluid ingestion). The guidelines evolved accordingly. By 1996, guidelines stated, "individuals should be encouraged to consume the maximal amount of fluids during exercise that can be tolerated without gastrointestinal discomfort up to a rate equal to that lost from sweating." This may have been interpreted by some as "to drink as much as tolerable." Since then the American College of Sports Medicine has reworded the advice to "The goal of drinking during exercise is to prevent excessive dehydration (>2% BW loss from water deficit) and excessive changes in electrolyte balance to avert compromised exercise performance. The amount and rate of fluid

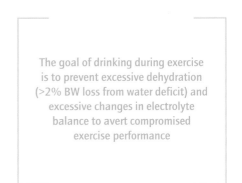

The goal of drinking during exercise is to prevent excessive dehydration (>2% BW loss from water deficit) and excessive changes in electrolyte balance to avert compromised exercise performance

replacement depends upon the individual sweating rate, exercise duration, and opportunities to drink" (Sawka et al. 2007a). Regular measurements of body weight can help to determine the sweat losses. Table 1 gives an overview of estimated sweat rates for persons with different body weights and sweat rates.

Important to have consistency in placement of text and Table or Figure number? See below. Always on top or always on the bottom? See below. I have not checked this throughout and perhaps it is not important.

Table 1: Estimated weight losses (as % body weight) while running a marathon at different paces and ingesting different amounts of fluid. The combinations highlighted in orange are either insufficient fluid intake (resulting in weight loss of >3%) or excessive fluid intake (weight gain).

Marathon time (h)		05:00	04:30	04:00	03:30	03:00
Pace (min·mile)		11:30	10:20	09:12	08:00	06:55
Pace (km·h)		8.4	9.4	10.6	12.1	14.1
Sweat rate (Liters ·h)		0.4	0.5	0.6	0.8	1
Person 50 kg	0.0	-4.0%	-4.5%	-4.8%	-5.6%	-6.0%
	0.2	-2.0%	-2.7%	-3.2%	-4.2%	-4.8%
	0.4	0.0%	-0.9%	-1.6%	-2.8%	-3.6%
	0.6	2.0%	0.9%	0.0%	-1.4%	-2.4%
	0.8	4.0%	2.7%	1.6%	0.0%	-1.2%
	1.0	6.0%	4.5%	3.2%	1.4%	0.0%
Person 65 kg	0.0	-3.1%	-3.5%	-3.7%	-4.3%	-4.6%
	0.2	-1.5%	-2.1%	-2.5%	-3.2%	-3.7%
	0.4	0.0%	-0.7%	-1.2%	-2.2%	-2.8%
	0.6	1.5%	0.7%	0.0%	-1.1%	-1.8%
	0.8	3.1%	2.1%	1.2%	0.0%	-0.9%
	1.0	4.6%	3.5%	2.5%	1.1%	0.0%
Person 80 kg	0.0	-2.5%	-2.8%	-3.0%	-3.5%	-3.8%
	0.2	-1.3%	-1.7%	-2.0%	-2.6%	-3.0%
	0.4	0.0%	-0.6%	-1.0%	-1.8%	-2.3%
	0.6	1.3%	0.6%	0.0%	-0.9%	-1.5%
	0.8	2.5%	1.7%	1.0%	0.0%	-0.8%
	1.0	3.8%	2.8%	2.0%	0.9%	0.0%

Caffeine, creatine and glycerol

Caffeine has long been recognized as a diuretic. For this reason it has often been advised to avoid caffeine, especially before and during exercise. In the early studies relatively large doses of caffeine were used (>300mg). However, in more recent studies, in which smaller doses were used, caffeine did not promote dehydration at rest or during exercise. Based on the current evidence there is no reason to restrict caffeine intake at levels below 300 mg (Table 2).

Creatine is a supplement used by many strength athletes. The intake of creatine usually increases body mass because water is stored in the intracellular space. It has been argued that water is drawn from the vascular space and that creatine intake should be restricted. However, there is no evidence that creatine ingested in normal doses increases heat stress or decreases performance in hot conditions. Based on the current evidence an advice to restrict creatine intake has no foundation (Table 2).

Glycerol is a hyper hydrating agent that is sometimes used before competition. Glycerol increases the water storage and can, in some conditions, protect against heat stress. There are also a few studies that demonstrate performance benefits. However, taking glycerol is not very practical and can cause side effects. Relatively large amounts of glycerol would have to be ingested with very large amounts of water. Headaches are very common. For these reasons glycerol hyper hydration is not a very user friendly strategy (Table 2).

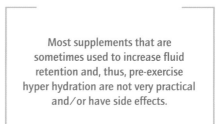

Most supplements that are sometimes used to increase fluid retention and, thus, pre-exercise hyper hydration are not very practical and/or have side effects.

Table 2: Supplements and their impact on hydration.

Supplement	Claim	Evidence
Caffeine	Caffeine is a diuretic and should be avoided before and during exercise	Caffeine ingested in moderate doses (up to 300mg) is not a diuretic and there is no reason to restrict caffeine intake at levels below 300 mg.
Creatine	Creatine increases water storage, removes water from the vascular space and increases heat stress	There is no evidence that creatine increases heat stress or decreases performance in hot conditions.
Glycerol	Glycerol is a hyper hydrating agent which increases water storage, reduces heat stress and improves exercise performance in the heat	Glycerol can result in increased water storage, reduced heat stress in extreme conditions and there are some reports of improved performance. Its use however, is impractical and can cause side effects.

Heat cramps

Cramps are common in athletes and seem to occur more, when the exercise is more prolonged, more intense and in hot conditions. Cramps are basically a form of motor unit hyperactivity and result in painful involuntary muscle contractions. Heat cramps are associated with large sweat (salt and water) losses. The difference between heat cramps and exercise associated cramps are subtle but the former can be confirmed if sodium replacement resolves the cramps. It seems to be possible to treat heat cramps quite effectively with sodium intake. Unfortunately, at present it is difficult to estimate sodium losses and therefore difficult to predict how much sodium athletes should take in extreme conditions. Sodium intake does not only have to take place during exercise. Sodium can simply be ingested with meals on the day before competition. Although the exact etiology of heat cramps is unknown and difficult to investigate, sodium deficits seem to play an important role in the development of cramps.

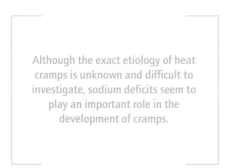

Although the exact etiology of heat cramps is unknown and difficult to investigate, sodium deficits seem to play an important role in the development of cramps.

Combining energy and fluid

Especially during prolonged exercise when carbohydrates reserves become depleted, carbohydrate intake, in addition to fluid intake, is important. However, it is known that with increasing carbohydrate intake (increasing carbohydrate concentration), the absorption of fluid may be impaired. Hence sports drinks are always a compromise between delivering energy and delivering fluid. Most sports drinks are in the 4-8% carbohydrate range where the impairment in fluid absorption is still acceptable. In the >10% range, however, it is generally thought that both gastric emptying and absorption of fluid are hampered even though it may result in a greater delivery of carbohydrate. We recently advised very high carbohydrate intakes for prolonged exercise in the region of 90 g·h (1.5 g·min). Interestingly, when such large amounts of carbohydrate were ingested in the form of glucose+fructose, the delivery of carbohydrate to the working muscle was improved (Figure 1) (Jeukendrup et al. 2006) and performance was increased 8% more than with a traditional sports drink containing one type of carbohydrate (Currell et al. 2008).

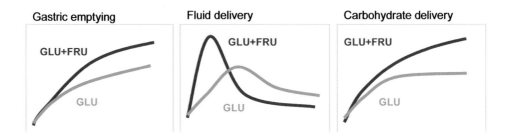

Figure 1: Multiple transportable carbohydrates such as fructose and glucose (GLU+FRU) appear to have faster gastric emptying, and result in greater fluid and carbohydrate delivery compared with a single carbohydrate (Glucose: GLU). Figure redrawn from (Jeukendrup et al. 2008; Jeukendrup et al. 2006).

Such large amounts of carbohydrate can only be delivered in concentrated carbohydrate solutions provided very large volumes of fluid would be consumed. For example, to ingest 90 g of carbohydrate per hour, one would have to drink 750 ml of a 12% carbohydrate solution or 1.5L of a 6% carbohydrate solution. Ingesting 1.5L·h⁻¹ is not always practical or even possible. Alternatively, one would have to resort to drinking a more concentrated solution. According to existing information this would reduce fluid delivery. However, in studies where stable isotopes were used to label water and study fluid delivery it was demonstrated that mixtures of glucose and fructose had a faster rate of gastric emptying and a superior fluid delivery compared with a single carbohydrate

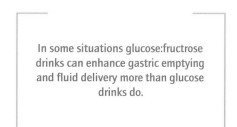

In some situations glucose:fructrose drinks can enhance gastric emptying and fluid delivery more than glucose drinks do.

(Figure 1). Therefore, in situations where both carbohydrate and fluid delivery are important and the exercise duration is >2h, it would be advisable to drink solutions with multiple transportable carbohydrates and ensure an intake of 60-90g·h⁻¹.

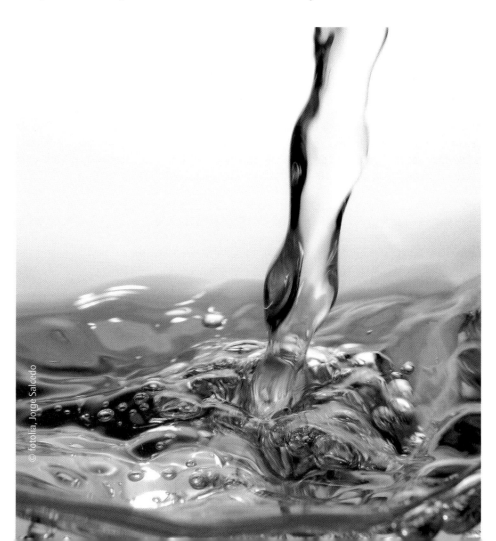

© fotolia, Jorge Salcedo

Chapter 6

Fat burning: how and why?

Asker Jeukendrup

> Although evidence for this is not available, it is appealing to think that an increased capacity to oxidize fat may aid those who want to lose weight and, in particular, body fat if used in combination with a negative energy balance.

Fat burning is a very popular and often used term among endurance athletes. There are fat burning workouts, fat burning nutrition supplements (fat burners), exercise machines in the gym have fat burning options and heart rate monitors tell you when you are in the fat burning zone. The term fat burning refers to the ability to oxidize (or burn) fat and use fat as a fuel instead of carbohydrate. Often fat burning is associated with weight loss, decreases in body fat and increases in lean body mass. However, it must be noted that such changes in body weight and body composition can only be achieved with a negative energy balance: you have to eat less calories than you expend, independent of the fuels you use! It is important to realize that increasing fat oxidation does not mean losing body fat or body weight! Here we will discuss the importance of fat burning and the most important factors influencing it as well as nutrition supplements that claim to increase fat burning.

The importance of fat metabolism

It is becoming increasingly clear that the ability to oxidize fat is important for both performance and health. It is also well established that well-trained endurance athletes have an increased capacity to oxidize fatty acids. This enables them to use fat as a fuel when carbohydrate stores become limited. In contrast, patients with obesity, insulin resistance and type II diabetes may have an impaired capacity to oxidize fat. As a result, fatty acids may be stored in the muscle and in other tissues. This accumulation of lipid in the muscle and its metabolites may interfere with the regulation of metabolism. Although evidence for this is not available it is appealing to think that an increased capacity to oxidize fat may aid those who want to lose weight and, in particular, body fat if used in combination with a negative energy balance.

Factors that affect fat oxidation

The factors that affect fat oxidation have been listed in Table 1 and will be discussed in the section below. Not all of these factors are equally important. They have, therefore, been ranked in order of importance based on the available evidence. Exercise intensity and diet are the most important factors and will be discussed first.

Table 1: Factors that affect substrate utilization

Exercise intensity	
Dietary intake	Especially carbohydrate intake has the potential to reduce fat oxidation
Exercise duration	The longer the duration the higher the fat oxidation
Mode of exercise	Running seems to increase fat oxidation more than cycling
Gender	Women oxidize slightly more fat than men
A very limited number of supplements that increase fat oxidation	Caffeine, green tea extracts
Altitude	Reduces fat oxidation
High environmental temperature	Reduces fat oxidation
Very cold conditions	Reduces fat oxidation

Exercise intensity

One of the most important factors that determine the rate of fat oxidation during exercise is the intensity. Although several studies have described the relationship between exercise intensity and fat oxidation, it was not until recently that this relationship was studied over a wide range of intensities (Achten et al. 2003b) (Figure 1). In absolute terms, findings showed that carbohydrate oxidation will increase proportionally with exercise intensity and that the rate of fat oxidation will initially increase but will decrease again at higher exercise intensities (Figure 1). Thus, while it is often claimed that you have to exercise at low intensities to oxidize fat, this is not necessarily true.

This exercise intensity (Fatmax) or "zone" may have importance for weight loss programs, health-related exercise programs, and endurance training.

In a series of recent studies we have defined the exercise intensity at which maximal fat oxidation is observed as *Fatmax*. In a group of trained individuals it was found that exercise at moderate intensity (62-63%VO_2max or 70-75%HRmax; (Figure 1) was the optimal intensity for fat oxidation, whereas it was around 50%VO_2max for less trained individuals (Achten et al. 2003b; Jeukendrup et al. 2005)). It is important to note that the inter-individual variation is very large. A trained person may have his maximal fat oxidation at 70%VO_2max or 45%VO_2max and the only way to really find out is to perform one of these *Fatmax* tests in the laboratory. However, in reality the exact exercise intensity at which fat oxidation peaks may not be that important because within 5-10% of this intensity (or 10-15 beats per minute), fat oxidation will be similarly high. It is only when the intensity is approximately 20% higher that fat oxidation will drop rapidly (Figure 1). This exercise intensity *(Fatmax)* or "zone" may have importance for weight loss programs, health-related exercise programs, and endurance training. However, very little research has been done to date.

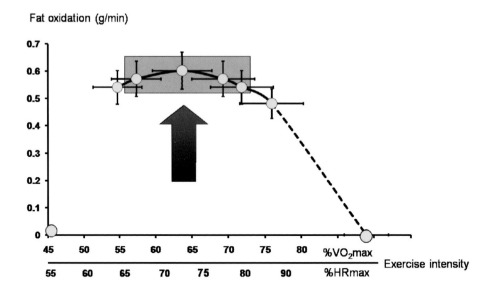

Figure 1: Exercise intensity (expressed as %HRmax and %VO₂max) and fat oxidation. Fat oxidation increases from low to moderate exercise intensities, peaks at Fatmax and decreases as the exercise intensity increases further. The grey area represents the fat zone: a range of exercise intensities where fat oxidation is high.

Dietary effect

The other important factor is diet. A diet high in carbohydrate will suppress fat oxidation and a diet low in carbohydrate will result in high fat oxidation rates. Ingesting carbohydrate in the hours before exercise will raise raise insulin production and subsequently suppress fat oxidation by up to about 35% (Achten et al. 2003a). This effect of insulin on fat oxidation may last as long as 6-8 hours after a meal which means that the highest fat oxidation rates can be achieved after an overnight fast. Exercise without breakfast has often been used by endurance athletes as a way to increase the fat oxidative capacity of the muscle. Recently a study was performed at the University of Leuven in Belgium in which they investigated the effect of an endurance training program (6 wk, 3 day·wk⁻¹, 1–2 h) (De Bock et al. 2008). The participants trained either in the fasted or in the carbohydrate fed state. The investigators observed a decrease in muscle glycogen use and an increase in the activity of various enzymes involved in fat metabolism after training in the fasted state. However, fat oxidation during exercise was the same in both groups. It is possible, though, that there are small but significant changes in fat metabolism after fasted training. In this study changes in fat oxidation might have been masked by the fact that these subjects received carbohydrate during their experimental trials. Research has shown that training after an overnight fast may reduce the exercise capacity. Therefore, it may only be suitable for low to moderate intensity exercise sessions. The efficacy of such training for weight reduction is also not known.

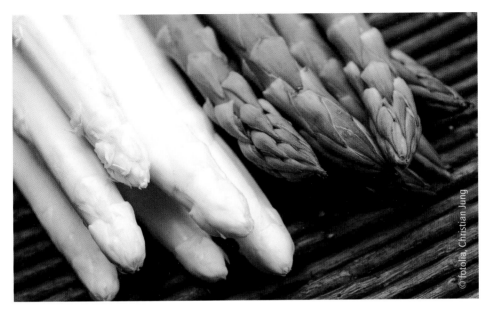

© fotolia, Christian Jung

Duration of exercise

It has been long established that fat oxidation becomes an increasingly important fuel as exercise progresses. During ultra-endurance exercise fat oxidation can reach peaks of 1 g/min although fat oxidation may be reduced if carbohydrate is ingested before or during exercise. In terms of weight loss, the duration of exercise may be one of the key factors as it is also the most effective way to increase energy expenditure.

The mode of exercise

The choice of exercise also has an effect on fat oxidation. Fat oxidation has been shown to be higher for a given oxygen uptake during walking and running compared with cycling (Achten et al. 2003c). The exact reason for this is not known though it has been suggested that it is related to the greater power output per muscle fiber in cycling compared to running.

Gender differences

Although some studies in the literature have found no gender differences in metabolism, the majority of studies now indicate higher rates of fat oxidation in women compared with men. In a study in which 150 men and 150 women were compared over a wide range of exercise intensities, it was demonstrated that the women had higher rates of fat oxidation over the entire range of intensities and fat oxidation peaked at a slightly higher intensity (Venables et al. 2005). The differences are small, however, and may not be of great physiological significance.

Environment

Environmental conditions can also influence substrate utilization. It is known that exercise in a hot environment will increase glycogen use and reduce fat oxidation. This can also be observed at high altitude. Similarly when it is extremely cold carbohydrate metabolism will be stimulated at the expense of fat metabolism, especially when shivering occurs.

Exercise training

At present, the only effective way to increase fat oxidation during exercise is to perform regular physical activity. This will up regulate the enzymes of the fat oxidation pathways and will increase mitochondrial mass and blood flow, all of which enable higher rates of fat oxidation. Research has shown that as little as 4 weeks of regular exercise (3 times per week 30-60 min) can increase fat oxidation rates and cause enzymatic changes (Holloszy et al. 1984). Too little information is available to draw any conclusions about the optimal training program to achieve these effects.

Exercise programs to lose weight or body fat

The optimal exercise type, intensity, and duration for weight loss are still unclear. Current recommendations are focused mainly on increasing energy expenditure and participation in exercise. Finding the optimal intensity for fat oxidation might aid in losing weight (fat loss) and support weight maintenance, but evidence for this is currently lacking. It is also important to realize that the amount of fat oxidized during exercise is actually small. Fat oxidation rates are, on average, 0.5 g·min at the optimal exercise intensity which means that more than 33 hours of exercise would be required to oxidize 1 kg of fat mass. Walking or running activity around 50-65% VO_2max seems to be an optimal intensity to oxidize fat. The duration of exercise plays a crucial role as this dictates in large art the energy expenditure and fat oxidation increases with increasing duration of exercise. Of course this also has the potential to increase daily energy expenditure. If exercise is the only intervention used, the main goal is usually to increase energy expenditure and reduce body fat. When combined with a diet program, however, it is mainly used to counteract the decrease in fat oxidation often seen after weight loss (Astrup 1993).

Nutrition supplements

There are many nutrition supplements on the market that claim to increase fat oxidation. These supplements include caffeine, carnitine, hydroxycitric acid (HCA), chromium, conjugated linoleic acid (CLA), guarana, citrus aurantium, Asian ginseng, cayenne pepper, coleus forskholii, glucomannan, green tea, psyllium and pyruvate. (A selection of supplements is listed in Table 2.) With few exceptions, there is little or no evidence that these particular supplements actually increase fat oxidation during exercise (Jeukendrup et al. 2004). We will discuss three supplements below. The rest is summarized in the table.

> The only highly effective way to increase fat oxidation is through exercise training, although it is still unclear what the best training regimen is to get the largest improvements.

Carnitine

Carnitine is one of the most popular fat burners. It has been around for a long time and became very popular in the 90s after the Italian football team won the world champion and revealed that they had used carnitine. Carnitine is a substance produced by the body but also obtained via daily food intake. It is found mostly in meat and plays a crucial role in fat metabolism. Carnitine is responsible for the transport of fats into the mitochondria (the power plants in the cells that provide the muscle with the energy to contract). Patients who cannot synthesize carnitine are, therefore, unable to use fat as a fuel and must rely solely on carbohydrate. The entire theory that carnitine supplementation helps fat metabolism is based on the premise that when you ingest carnitine it then enters the muscle and the concentration of carnitine in the muscle increases. Studies in the 90s showed, however, that even with a large dose of carnitine, the muscle carnitine concentration is unaffected. Thus, carnitine cannot expect to have an effect on fat metabolism. Scientists lost interest in carnitine though athletes were still buying carnitine! Recently however, there is some renewed interest in carnitine. Professor Paul Greenhaff and his coworkers at the University of Nottingham showed that IF you can increase the muscle carnitine, this can increase fat metabolism. They increased muscle carnitine by simultaneously increasing the insulin concentration and providing carnitine. While it is possible that carnitine may have some effect if used in combination with carbohydrate, in the long term, it is now too early to draw any conclusions. The fact remains that most studies have not observed any effects of carnitine.

Green tea or green tea extracts

Green tea has many suggested medicinal properties and there is actually some evidence that is does protect against various diseases. More recently research has focused on its effects on fat metabolism and although 90% of the research is on animals, and not on humans, the results are promising. We recently showed that ingesting a green tea extract the night before and an hour before a 30 min cycling bout increased fat metabolism by 20% (Venables et al. 2008). The green tea extract contains mainly Epogalocatechin gallate or EGCG, the active ingredient in green tea. EGCG is one of most powerful polyphenols with anti-oxidant properties. It can result in increased the activity of the enzyme responsible for the breakdown of catecholamines (adrenaline and noradrenaline). This in turn may result in higher concentrations of catecholamines and stimulation of lipolysis making more fatty acids available for oxidation. There is also some evidence that EGCG increases metabolic rate suggesting that it could help with weight loss. The green tea extract contains the active ingredient in a concentrated form. The dose used, which produced the 20% improvement in fat metabolism, was fairly large. It would equate to drinking a liter of green tea. At present we are studying the effects of smaller doses of green tea.

Caffeine

Caffeine is often associated with increased fat metabolism. However, whether caffeine actually has this effect depends on the exercise type and the dose of caffeine. Effects on fat metabolism are typically seen at lower intensities of exercise and with relatively low doses of caffeine. At high doses of caffeine and at higher intensities of exercise, carbohydrate metabolism may be stimulated and fat metabolism may even be suppressed. Several "fat burners" contain at least some caffeine.

Does a cup of coffee with breakfast work? Probably not a lot! The reason for that is that a breakfast typically contains some carbohydrate. This will cause the hormone insulin to be released which in turn will suppress fat metabolism. So although caffeine may stimulate fat metabolism a little, this effect would be completely overruled by insulin.

In fact, this is the case for all supplements. Increased fat metabolism can probably only be observed in the morning, after an overnight fast and before breakfast. Therefore there is probably no easy option! You still have to exercise and you may have to do this without breakfast in order to stimulate fat metabolism. Fat burning exercise sessions can have a place in a weekly training schedule but it is probably not a good idea to do too many of these sessions in one week.

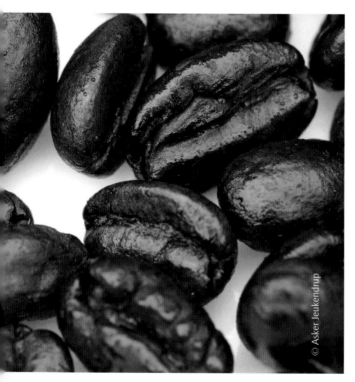

© Asker Jeukendrup

Summary

Higher fat oxidation rates during exercise generally reflect a good training status whereas low fat oxidation rates might be related to obesity and insulin resistance. Fat oxidation peaks on average at moderate exercise intensities, 50-65%VO_2max, depending on the training status of the individuals (Achten et al. 2003b; Venables et al. 2005). The rate of fat oxidation increases with increasing exercise duration but is suppressed by carbohydrate intake. Fat oxidation is slightly higher in women than in men. Also altitude and hot (or very cold) environmental conditions can increase carbohydrate and reduce fat oxidation. Many supplements claim to improve fat oxidation but most supplements are ineffective.

The only highly effective way to increase fat oxidation is through exercise training, although it is still unclear what the best training regimen is to get the largest improvements. Finally, it is important to note that there is a very large inter-individual variation in fat oxidation which is only partially explained by the factors mentioned above. This means that although certain factors can influence fat oxidation, their exact influence on one's fat oxidation rate is highly individual and cannot be predicted.

Table 2: Nutrition supplements and the scientific evidence that the supplement increases fat metabolism

Nutrition supplement	Evidence	Fat burning properties (claims)
Caffeine	○ ○ ● ● ●	Caffeine stimulates lipolysis and the mobilization of FAs. These actions might occur indirectly by increasing the circulating catecholamine levels or directly by antagonizing adenosine receptors that normally inhibit hormone-sensitive lipase and FA oxidation. In some, but not all conditions, this can result in increased fat oxidation.
Carnitine	○ ○ ○ ● ●	Carnitine is essential for fat oxidation as it is needed to transport fatty acids into the mitochondria. Studies have shown that carnitine supplementation may not result in increased muscle carnitine supplementation. Therefore, it is not surprising that no effects on fat oxidation have been found. Nevertheless, it is one of the supplements that is aggressively marketed as a fat burner. New studies may provide new insights.
Cayenne pepper (Capsaicin)	○ ○ ○ ● ●	Cayenne pepper has been used as a medicine for centuries, and has recently gained attention as a possible fat burning supplement. Cayenne contains capsaicin, which may help increase metabolic rate and stimulate circulation.
Chromium	○ ○ ○ ● ●	Chromium was a very popular supplement a few years ago and was associated with insulin sensitivity and fat burning. There is no evidence that chromium has any effect on fat metabolism.
Citrus aurantium	○ ○ ○ ● ●	Citrus aurantium (from bitter orange) contains five adrenergic amines including synephrine and tyramine, which stimulate the beta-3 cell receptors, stimulating lipolysis.

45

Coleus forskholii (Forskolin)	● ● ● ● ●	Coleus forskholii is an ancient herb that has gained attention lately as a possible fat burner.extract called Forskolin, present in Coleus, has been found to be beneficial in its ability to burn fat. Forskolin activates adenylate cyclase, which, in turn, triggers an increase in cyclic adenosine monophosphate (cAMP). This increase in cAMP turns on the system responsible for the release of fat from its stores.
Conjugated linoleic acid (CLA)	● ● ● ● ●	Fatty acids that have been linked with special properties (especially antioxidant properties) but have also been linked to increases in fat metabolism. Evidence is weak.
Guarana	● ● ● ● ●	The active constituent of guarana, guaranine, is nearly identical to caffeine and is likely to have similar properties. There is far less research with guaranine compared to research with caffeine.
Ginseng (Asian or Panax)	● ● ● ● ●	Asian ginseng (Panax ginseng) has been a part of Chinese medicine for over 2,000 years and was traditionally used to improve mental and physical vitality. Evidence for fat burning properties is lacking.
Glucomannan	● ● ● ● ●	Glucomannan is a dietary fiber derived from the Konjac plant of South East Asia. It is included in fat burning supplements probably because of its potential effect on appetite (food intake). The fiber itself has no effect on fat metabolism.
Green tea	● ● ● ● ●	The active constituents in green tea are the polyphenols, particularly the catechin, epigallocatechin gallate (EGCG). However, green tea also contains caffeine. A recent study showed that fat oxidation during exercise increased by about 20%.
Hydroxycitric acid (HCA)	● ● ● ● ●	HCA is a derivative of citric acid that is found in a variety of tropical plants. There is no evidence that it has any effect on fat metabolism
Pyruvate	● ● ● ● ●	Pyruvate is an intermediate of carbohydrate metabolism and as such it is difficult to see

		exactly how pyruvate intake could increase fat oxidation. Nevertheless, this is one of the claims often made.
Psyllium	• • • • •	Psyllium is a soluble fiber that comes from the small reddish black seeds of the Plantago Psyllium plant. Like glucomannan, psyllium is probably marketed as a fat burner because of its potential effect on appetite (food intake). However, the fiber itself has no effects on fat metabolism.
Tyrosine	• • • • •	L-tyrosine is a nonessential amino acid that serves as a precursor to catecholamines. The assumption is that more tyrosine results in chronically elevated catecholamine concentrations and increased lipolysis. There is no evidence to support this.

The scientific evidence is indicated with green dots.

•	One dot means limited to no evidence
• •	Two dot means limited evidence
• • •	Evidence
• • • •	Strong evidence
• • • • •	Very strong evidence

Chapter 7

Nutrition for recovery

Louise Burke

It is one thing to perform well in a single training session or event. Most athletes need to be able to bounce back for more – for the next training session, the semi-final, or the next match in the tournament. Their sporting success will ultimately depend on their ability to manage their recovery needs. Recovery involves a variety of issues and a range of strategies. Questions that the athlete should ask are:

- What needs to be recovered after this session?
- What nutrients will promote this recovery and how much do I need?
- What foods and drinks are suitable to provide these nutrients?

The answers will vary according to the athlete, the event and their overall nutrition goals.

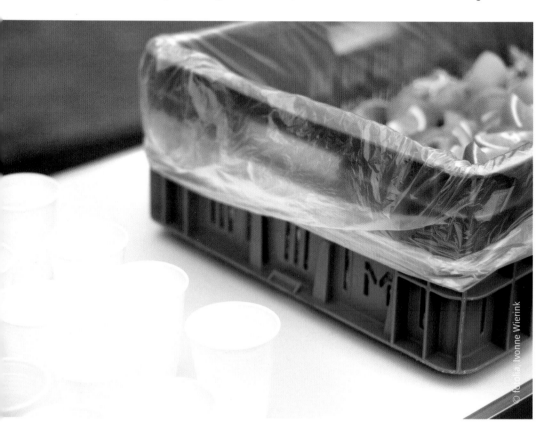

© Fotolia, Ivonne Wierink

Refueling

Lengthy workouts or sessions of repeated high intensity exercise will deplete muscle fuel (glycogen) stores. The two most important factors in restoring fuel levels are carbohydrate intake and time. Glycogen is stored at a relatively slow rate – it can take 24 hours to fill empty fuel tanks. But this also depends on having a supply of carbohydrate from foods or drinks to synthesize into glycogen. How much you need to consume will depend on the level of depletion you started from and what you need for the next session. Daily carbohydrate targets set by sports nutrition experts can provide some ball park targets. Table 1 in Chapter 2 summarizes these, and shows a range from 3-5 g of carbohydrate per kg body mass for a recreational jogger who has light fuel requirements for daily workouts of 30-60 minutes to 10-12 g·kg^{-1} BM for a Tour de France cyclist who is refueling between 4-8 hour stages. These should be considered a starting point and each athlete should experiment to find what works for his or her own needs and goals.

Studies of muscle cells show that they restore glycogen at a slightly higher rate in the couple of hours after an exercise session is over. Many people have made a big deal of this fact, describing it as a "window of opportunity" for refueling. However, as stated before, the most important factor in opening a window for refueling is a carbohydrate supply. In fact, some sports nutritionists prefer the message that effective refueling doesn't occur until the athlete consumes carbohydrate-rich foods and drinks after the workout or event. If there is plenty of time until the next session (for example, more than 8-24 hours), it doesn't matter if an hour or two is wasted before refueling kicks in. However, when time is short between fuel-demanding events, it makes sense to start refueling as soon as possible. The challenge may be to get home to a carbohydrate-rich snack or meal or to have a supply of suitable carbohydrate-rich drinks and foods handy to the field of training or competition. The immediate target should be around 1 g of carbohydrate per kg BM, repeated every hour until meal patterns take over the achievement of daily fuel needs.

> It if often said that there is a "window of opportunity" for refueling. However, the most important factor in opening a window for refueling is a carbohydrate supply.

There has been some interest in whether some carbohydrate-rich foods and snacks are better than others for refueling. One study showed that foods with a moderate-high glycemic index (GI) such as bread, flaky breakfast cereals, rice and most fruits/juices are more effective in promoting glycogen storage than foods with a low GI (e.g. beans, lentils, porridge). However, it is probably more important to think about practical factors such as whether foods and drinks are well-liked and available, and the nutritional value they supply. As we will see below, protein, electrolytes and fluid may also be needed for a full recovery, and it will be a clever plan to choose food sources that can supply all nutrient needs at once. In addition, the athlete needs to consider recovery eating after exercise as part of their total nutritional plan. It doesn't make sense if you are on an energy limit to blow your daily budget by eating large amounts of high fat/high kilojoule carbohydrates, or to neglect this as an opportunity to satisfy daily needs of vitamins, minerals and other health-promoting food components. Athletes who can mix and match foods to balance a number of goals will get the best from their recovery eating.

Once recovery eating is started, how should it be spread over the day? Most studies show that over a full day of recovery it doesn't appear to matter whether the muscle receives its carbohydrate supply in big meals or as a number of small snacks—at least as far as glycogen storage is concerned. As long as you can eat your way through your total carbohydrate needs each day (and have considered the benefits of an early start after the exercise session), the timing details are up to you. For some people, a 'grazing' pattern is less filling and more fun. However, other athletes do not have access to food or the opportunities to eat it all day and for them a routine of larger meals may be more suitable.

Rehydration

Even where an athlete has consumed fluid before and during an exercise session, it is likely that they will still finish the session with some degree of dehydration. Ideally, the athlete should aim to fully restore fluid losses after a workout or event in time for the next. This is difficult in situations where the fluid deficit is more than 2% of body mass and the interval between sessions is less than 6 to 8 hours. In normal circumstances, our thirst and urine losses allow us to do a good job in helping us replace fluid losses and maintain fluid balance from day to day. However, under acute situations of stress such as prolonged exercise, or a sudden change in temperature and altitude, thirst may not be a sufficient stimulus for maintaining fluid balance. This is where a fluid plan can be useful. This plan needs to consider the volume, the timing and the type of fluids (see also Chapter 5).

As is the case for fluids consumed during exercise, recovery drinks need to taste good so that you will be motivated to consume them. However, simply drinking a volume of fluid equal to the fluid deficit achieved over the session (roughly speaking, your weight change) won't fully restore fluid balance. After all, we are likely to keep sweating and producing urine during the next hours. Depending on factors such as the type and timing of what we consume, we may be good at retaining this fluid or we may waste a lot in unnecessary pit stops. Typically, a volume equal to 125-150% of the post-exercise fluid deficit must be drunk to compensate for these ongoing losses and ensure that fluid balance is restored over the first 4 to 6 h of recovery. This means that an athlete who is a kilogram lighter after a workout will need to drink 1250-1500 ml of fluid over the next hours to rehydrate fully. However, when sweat losses are large we also need to replace the electrolytes, particularly sodium ("salt") lost in sweat, to allow fluids to be retained and re-equilibrated into body fluid

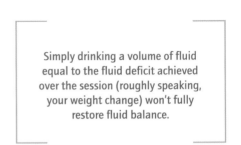
Simply drinking a volume of fluid equal to the fluid deficit achieved over the session (roughly speaking, your weight change) won't fully restore fluid balance.

compartments. Salt may be consumed in the form of high-electrolyte drinks, such as the Oral Rehydration Solutions produced for use in clinical cases of dehydration or diarrhea or special higher salt ("endurance") brands of sports drinks. Alternatively, salt may be consumed in the foods consumed in recovery meals and snacks, or added to the meal.

Repair and adaptation

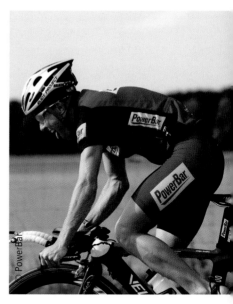

The repair and adaptation desired after many types of exercise relies on the manufacture of new proteins. The stimulus of exercise dictates which proteins are manufactured. For example, resistance exercise stimulates the synthesis of new structural proteins to make the muscle bigger and stronger. Endurance exercise promotes the synthesis of proteins that help the muscle be better at such exercise – for example enzymes that promote the use of fat as an exercise fuel, or transporters that help the muscle absorb glucose from the bloodstream, or fat into the mitochondria where it is oxidized. Protein synthesis increases in the hours after this exercise is undertaken, and new research shows that better repair and adaptation to a workout or an event may occur if the athlete consumes a source of high quality protein in this recovery phase. These ideas are covered in greater detail in Chapters 9 and 11. For the moment, we will just remember the value of incorporating protein into the meals and snacks following the key training sessions from which adaptation and repair is desired. It appears that when high quality proteins sources are chosen, especially animal foods such as dairy foods, meat and eggs, only small amounts are required to achieve good effects. As little as 10 g of protein achieves a worthwhile stimulation of protein synthesis while the effect is maxed out with a serving of 20-25 g of protein. This may be easily found in "main meals" featuring meat/fish/chicken, so the athlete who organizes training routines to finish just before normal meals may already be covered. However, Table 1 shows how protein can also be provided by lighter meals and snacks.

> Amounts of protein relevant for protein synthesis (10-25g) may be easily found in "main meals" featuring meat/fish/chicken, so the athlete who organizes training routines to finish just before normal meals may already be covered.

Staying healthy

Staying healthy and injury free is a key goal in sport. One of the downsides of training hard to promote maximal adaptation is that you put your immune system and bones under stress. Recovery eating should, therefore, take into account the factors that help immune function and other systems that keep us healthy and injury free. This is a less developed area of recovery nutrition. At this stage we can't offer absolute rules of what is needed. However, we can offer a couple of general guidelines:

- Your immune system functions best when carbohydrate is available. Generally, strenuous exercise suppresses immune function and gives bugs their own "window of opportunity." After a workout when you are most vulnerable to attack. Making sure that you were well fueled before, during and after a session helps to reduce the immune-suppressing effect of strenuous exercise on your immune system (see also Chapters 15 and 16).
- Adequate energy is important for your immune system and bone health. Therefore, it makes sense to avoid energy restriction during periods of key training or competition. This can occur because you are deliberately trying to lose weight/body fat or because you are unaware of or disorganized in meeting your energy and fuel needs The higher your needs are, the more important it is to have a plan rather than leaving it to good luck.
- Other nutrients may be important for the immune system and bones in terms of both quantity and timing. It makes sense to choose nutrient-rich foods in your general diet and for recovery eating.
- New research may uncover benefits of consuming probiotics/prebiotics, getting plenty of Vitamin D and other nutritional strategies to improve the immune system and to promote bone health of athletes in heavy training.

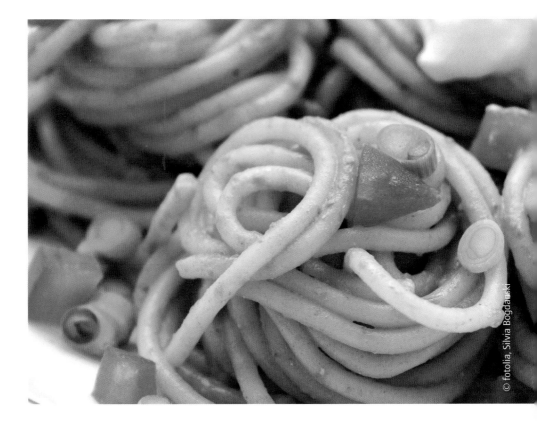

© fotolia, Silvia Bogdanski

Table 1: Ideas for recovery snacks and light meals

Note that these choices provide:
- 50 g carbohydrate
- At least 10 g protein

Many also provide a good source of:
- sodium and fluid
- vitamins, minerals and other health-promoting food components

- 250-350 ml of liquid meal supplement (e.g. Power bar Protein Plus or Recovery drink)
- 250-350 ml of milk shake or fruit smoothie
- 500 ml flavored low fat milk
- 60 g (1.5-2 cups) breakfast cereal with 1/2 cup milk
- 1 sandwiche with cheese/meat/chicken filling, and 1 large piece of fruit or 300 ml sports drink
- 1 cup of fruit salad with 200 g carton fruit-flavored yoghurt or custard
- 200 g carton fruit-flavored yoghurt or 300 ml flavored milk and 30-35 g cereal bar
- 2 crumpets or English muffins with thick spread of peanut butter or 2 slices of cheese
- 200 g (cup or small tin) of baked beans on 2 slices of toast
- 250 g (large) baked potato with cottage cheese or grated cheese filling
- 150 g thick crust pizza with meat/chicken/seafood topping

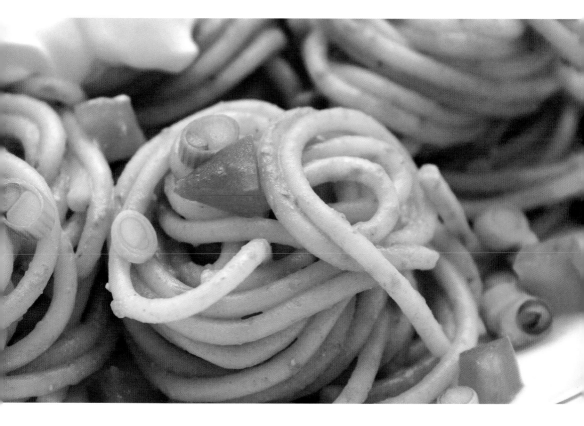

Chapter 8

Nutrition, sleep and recovery

Shona L. Halson

Ensuring athletes achieve an appropriate quality and/or quantity of sleep may have significant implications on performance and recovery and reduce the risk of developing overreaching or overtraining. Indeed, sleep is often suggested to be the single best recovery strategy available to elite athletes. A number of nutritional factors which have been suggested to improve sleep include: valerian, melatonin, tryptophan, a high glycemic index diet before bedtime and maintaining a balanced and healthy diet. Other factors like the consumption of alcohol and caffeine and hyper-hydration may disturb sleep.

Functions of sleep

The fundamental question of *why* humans require sleep is largely unanswered. Despite this, scientists are providing increased information regarding how humans sleep. As the duration and timing of sleep are tightly regulated, it is assumed that sleep serves a number of important psychological and physiological functions. It is probable, that sleep has multiple functions across a diverse range of physical and cognitive aspects and that these functions are strongly interrelated.

> Sleep disturbances may have an influence on athletic performance, particularly if they occur over a prolonged period. Identifying athletes who are experiencing poor sleep is critical as it may lead to overtraining, illness or precipitate injury.

Sleep and exercise performance

While the exact function of sleep may not be clear, the effects of sleep deprivation on exercise performance are somewhat clearer. A summary of postulated effects of sleep loss on various exercise tasks is summarized in Table 1. Studies have demonstrated changes in exercise performance following partial sleep deprivation. Sinnerton and Reilly (1992) measured eight swimmers following 2.5 hours of sleep per night over 4 nights. No effect of sleep loss was observed when investigating back and grip strength, lung function or swimming performance. However, mood state was significantly altered with increases in depression, tension, confusion, fatigue and anger and decreases in vigor. Partial sleep deprivation, in the form of three nights of sleep loss followed by one night of recovery

(Reilly and Deykin 1983), resulted in minimal changes in gross motor functions (muscle strength, lung power and endurance performance) while psychomotor function significantly declined, most of which was evident after only one night of sleep loss. Similar effects on sleep have been observed in both males and females.

Sustained exercise may be more affected than single maximal efforts and thus longer sub maximal exercise tasks may be affected following sleep deprivation (Reilly and Edwards 2007).

In terms of cognitive performance, sleep supplementation in the form of napping has been shown to have a positive influence on cognitive tasks. Naps can markedly reduce sleepiness and can be beneficial when learning skills, strategy or tactics (Postolache and Oren 2005).

Table 1: A taxonomy of sports and recreational activities affected by sleep loss (Reilly and Edwards 2007)

Characteristics	Sports	Effects
Low aerobic	Road cycling, aiming sports	Increased errors
Moderate aerobic, High concentration	Team sports	Decreased decision making
High aerobic	Running 3000m, swimming 400m	Marginal
Aerobic/ anaerobic	Swimming, middle distance running	Decreased power
Anaerobic	Sprints, power events	Marginal
Repeat anaerobic	Jumping events, weight-training	Increased fatigue

Sleep and recovery

Findings suggest that the recuperative and restorative effects of sleep are necessary and beneficial for athletic recovery. In particular, impairments in the immune and endocrine system that may result from sleep deprivation may impair the recovery process and hence adaptation to training (Reilly and Edwards 2007). Appropriate sleep quality and quantity is anecdotally reported to be the single best recovery strategy available to elite athletes. Alternatively, appropriate recovery strategies may aid sleep in several ways. Recovery strategies such as hydrotherapy may influence skin temperature which, as discussed in a later section, may initiate sleep onset. Further, appropriate recovery may result in a decrease in inflammation and pain, which may increase the ability to sleep, particularly in recently injured athletes.

Nutritional factors that may enhance sleep

There are a number of nutritional substances that have been traditionally associated with promoting sleep. Research has recently begun to investigate their effectiveness as a substitute for pharmacological intervention.

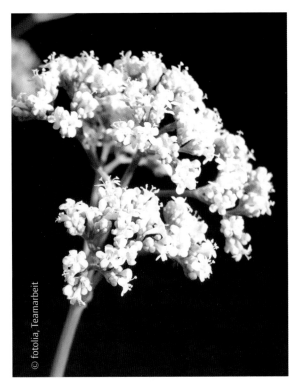

© fotolia, Teamarbeit

Valerian

Valerian *(Valeriana officinalis)*, or valerian root, is a flowering plant and is commonly used to treat insomnia and anxiety. It is the most commonly used herbal product to induce sleep in both the USA and Europe (Bent et al., 2006). In a recent systematic review and meta-analysis of the efficacy of valerian for improving sleep quality, Bent et al. (2006) suggest that valerian might improve sleep without producing side-effects. Of the 16 studies assessed there were a number of methodological issues which limited the ability to draw firm conclusions. However, results suggested that valerian can improve sleep. There were also trends for decreasing subjective sleep onset latency (SOL; is the length of time that it takes to accomplish the transition from full wakefulness to sleep).

Other sedative herbs

Kava is an extract from the root of *Piper methysticum*, a Polynesian plant, and has been used for its sedative effects. Research has shown some positive anti-anxiety effects. However, it has been withdrawn from the market in a number of countries due to adverse side-effects. Other compounds suggested to have sedative effects include: Melissa, Passion flower and Hops. Currently, with the exception of the plant Melissa (also known as lemon balm), there is a lack of scientific evidence regarding their usefulness.

Tryptophan

Tryptophan is an essential amino acid which is converted to serotonin (5-hydroxytryptamine: 5-HT) in the brain. The conversion occurs when the ratio of free- tryptophan to branched-chain amino acids (f-TRP: BCAA) is increased, resulting in an increase in brain tryptophan. Through 5-Hydroxytophan, free-tryptophan is converted to serotonin, which, in turn, is converted to melatonin.

L-tryptophan ingestion has previously been shown to decrease SOL by 45% (Hartmann 1982). Arnulf et al (2002) reported increased sleep fragmentation, increased sleep REM latency and increased REM density following daytime tryptophan depletion. Thus lowering plasma *f-TRP can have opposing effects on sleep to that of increasing plasma f-TRP.*

The results of the above studies suggest that the intake of tryptophan may improve sleep onset latency and alter rapid eye movement sleep onset latency. Tryptophancontaining foods include: milk, meat, fish, poultry, eggs, beans, peanuts, cheese and leafy green vegetables. Further research is required to accurately prescribe timing and dosage of tryptophan.

High glycemic index meals

Another possible method of altering serotonin is through the intake of high glycemic index (GI) meals. High GI carbohydrates may increase f-TRP: BCAA, facilitated through the release of insulin, which promotes the uptake of BCAA into the muscle. As plasma BCAA's decrease, the f-TRP:BCAA ratio increases, resulting in an increase in brain f-TRP and serotonin (Afaghi et al. 2007). Alternatively, high GI meals may reduce free fatty acids (FFA's), also through the release of insulin. In a recent study, meals with the same energy content were provided to subjects, with the only difference being the glycemic index of 200g of steamed rice (Mahatma long grain rice-GI=50 (low) or Jasmine aromatic long grain rice- GI=109 (high)) (Afaghi et al. 2007). High GI meals were provided at 1 and 4 hours prior to bedtime and low GI meals were consumed 4 hours prior to bedtime. The results showed that the high GI meal provided 4 hours prior to bedtime shortened SOL by 48.6% when compared to the low GI meal. Furthermore, the high GI meal resulted in a shortened SOL (38.3%) when consumed 4 hours prior to bedtime when compared to consumption 1 hour prior to bedtime.

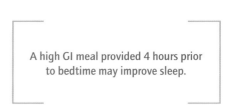

A high GI meal provided 4 hours prior to bedtime may improve sleep.

More extreme dietary conditions may result in more significant alterations in sleep. Ramadan, observed by millions of Muslims, involves abstaining from eating, drinking and smoking from dawn to sunset for a period of one month. In eight Muslim subjects assessed during Ramadan, there was a significant delay in sleep onset, which was associated with an increase in nocturnal body temperature (Roky et al. 2001). Slow wave sleep and REM sleep were also decreased, which may be related to increased cortisol concentrations and/or an increased body temperature (Roky et al. 2001). These results may have implications for athletes in weight-restricted sports and methods of improving sleep in these athletes may be necessary. Recommendations for enhancing sleep are included at the end of this chapter.

Melatonin

Melatonin (N-acetyl-5-methoxytryptamine) is a pineal hormone that is suggested to be associated with the control of circadian rhythms (Atkinson et al. 2003). As described earlier, melatonin is converted from serotonin and its precursor tryptophan. Melatonin also induces a hypothermic effect with reductions in core temperature ranging from 0.01-0.3°C. There are only a small number of studies that have investigated the use of melatonin in the treatment of insomnia. Generally, melatonin has been found to decrease subjective estimates of sleep latency and to increase total sleep time.

Nutritional factors that may decrease sleep

Alcohol

Due to the relatively fast metabolism of alcohol, the effects of alcohol on sleep can differ between the first and second half of the night. Research has demonstrated that although individuals fall asleep faster, sleep during the second half of the night can be interrupted with frequent wakings, increased dreaming and lower quality of sleep (Rundell et al. 1972).

> While some nutrients may enhance sleep, others, like alcohol and caffeine, can be detrimental to a good night's sleep.

Caffeine

Caffeine is considered a mild central nervous system stimulant and is the most commonly used methylxanthine. Caffeine can be found in a range of products, with coffee and tea being the most common sources. There is a widely held belief that caffeine may impair sleep, although individual differences in tolerance are commonly reported. It has been suggested that caffeine administered within two hours of bedtime can increase sleep latency, decrease slow wave sleep and decrease total sleep time. These effects can occur in doses of 100mg or greater. The negative influence of caffeine on sleep is of particular concern for those athletes who use relatively high doses of caffeine for performance enhancement, for events in the late afternoon/evening.

Hyper-hydration

Another nutritional factor involved with sleep quantity and quality may be hydration. In a recent survey of sleep habits of athletes at the Australian Institute of Sport, a major reason for sleep disturbances was getting up several times during the night to urinate. One reason for this is the need for rehydration following afternoon or evening training sessions or competition, possibly resulting in hyper-hydration in some individuals.

Other factors to enhance sleep

Skin warming

Sleep onset tends to occur when core body temperature is declining and sleep ends when it is rising. Prescription sleep medications, such as Temazepan and commercially available melatonin, result in vasodilation of distal skin regions. This in turn results in heat loss and a lowering of the core temperature which, in turn, initiates sleep onset.

Hydrotherapy

There is a small degree of scientific evidence to suggest that water therapy of some kind may elevate skin temperature and thus may result in enhanced sleep. Shortened sleep latency and increased sleepiness has been observed following warm baths and or/ foot baths that increased skin temperature (Horne and Shackell 1987; Sung and Tochihara 2000).

Other forms of hydrotherapy typically used to enhance athlete recovery will result in changes in skin and core temperature. Cold water immersion, contrast water therapy and hot water immersion (spa baths), all have the potential to change both skin and core temperature. While speculative, it is possible that the enhanced feelings of recovery and well-being typically experienced by athletes the day following hydrotherapy recovery may be, in part, related to enhanced sleep.

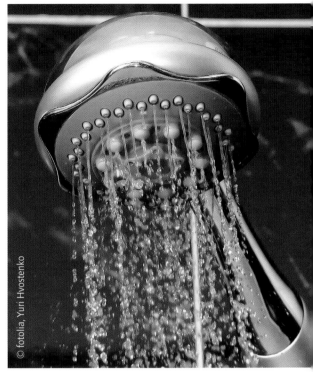

© fotolia, Yuri Hvostenko

Sleep hygiene

Sleep hygiene refers to behaviors that are believed to promote improved quality and quantity of sleep. Typically, this involves avoiding behaviors that interfere with sleep patterns and/or to engage in behaviors that promote good sleep. Table 2 includes a list of sleep hygiene recommendations.

Empirical evidence for the use of sleep hygiene recommendations as a treatment for insomnia is limited, mainly due to a lack of research and methodological limitations. However, poor sleep hygiene is generally not regarded as the primary cause of insomnia, although may contribute to it.

Recommendations

Based on the information presented above, a number of non-pharmacological methods may be effective for enhancing sleep. It is important to recognize that much of the sleep research has not been conducted on elite athletes; indeed, the majority of research has been on non-athletes. Therefore, until research has been conducted on elite athletes, these guidelines remain appropriate.

Table 2: Recommended non-pharmacological means for promoting sleep quality and / or quantity

Ensure appropriate recovery from training and competition (physical, nutritional and psychological)

Consume tryptophancontaining foods such as milk, meat, fish, poultry, eggs, beans, peanuts, cheese and leafy green vegetables

Consume a high glycemic index meal 4 hours before bedtime

Consume a balanced, healthy diet

Minimize alcohol intake prior to bedtime

Minimize caffeine intake prior to bedtime (individual tolerances do exist)

Proper fluid intake following completion of training/competition and before bedtime. For athletes who repeatedly wake at night to use the bathroom, hydration testing and fluid balance assessment may be useful to prescribe the right type and quantity of fluid for both the day and the recovery period.

Skin warming (in cool environmental conditions) can be achieved through warm/spa baths or hot footbaths before bed, warm blankets and wearing of socks

Skin cooling (in warm environmental conditions) can be achieved through cool showers and appropriate use of air-conditioning

Common sleep strategies:
- If you cannot sleep within 15 minutes, get out of bed and try another strategy.
- Eliminate the bedroom clock
- Avoid coffee, alcohol and nicotine
- Regularize the bedtime
- Be conscious of food choices and food intake
- Nap appropriately (for no more than 45 minutes and not late in the afternoon)

Explore techniques for muscle relaxation and cognitive relaxation

It is essential that athletes who sleep poorly seek medical advice to ensure there is no underlying medical condition which is causing disturbed sleep. Depression and anxiety are common causes of insomnia and it is vital that conditions such as these are treated appropriately.

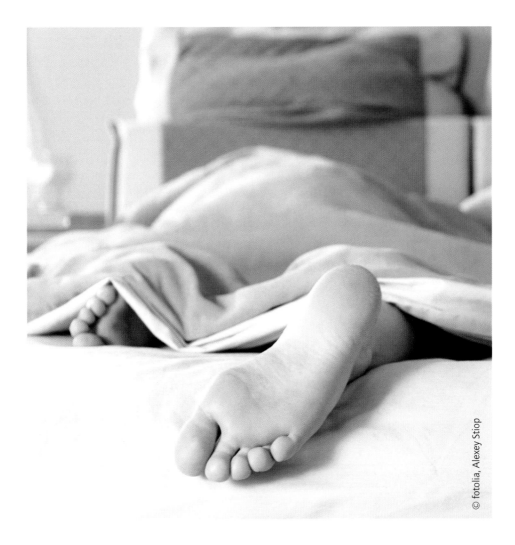

© fotolia, Alexey Stiop

Summary

There is limited scientific information regarding sleep requirements and characteristics in elite athletes. However, from the available evidence it appears that sleep disturbances may have an influence on athletic performance, particularly if they occur over a prolonged period. Identifying athletes who are experiencing poor sleep is critical as it may lead to overtraining, illness or precipitate injury. An awareness of the nutritional factors that may positively or negatively influence sleep may enable athletes to reap the full restorative benefits of good sleep. Adhering to sleep hygiene recommendations is another important step.

Chapter 9

Building muscle

Stuart Phillips and Mark Tarnopolsky

By far and away the most important factor for increasing muscle mass and strength is resistance exercise training. Even in a fasted state, resistance exercise training promotes the retention of protein. After a period of training there is an increase in muscle mass and strength.

General nutritional strategies

Nutrition can influence the response to resistance exercise training in multiple ways:

1. The total energy content of the diet must be sufficient to meet the needs of daily turnover and the energy cost of physical activity.

2. An adequate carbohydrate intake also enhances protein retention with the added benefit of maintaining glycogen stores for any endurance component of cycled training (> 4 g$\cdot$kg$^{-1}\cdot$d^{-1} for women; > 6 g$\cdot$kg$^{-1}\cdot$d^{-1} for men).

3. There is an increase in dietary protein requirements at the onset of resistance exercise training; however, the body adapts to this stress and, with time, the increase in protein requirements is attenuated. The *maximum* dietary protein requirement for an elite athlete performing weight training and/or endurance training would be 1.7 g$\cdot$kg$^{-1}\cdot$d^{-1}.

4. Finally, the timing of nutrient delivery around each of the training bouts is particularly important. Numerous studies have shown that the early provision of protein in the early period following resistance exercise can enhance protein retention. In addition, the inclusion of carbohydrate serves to suppress protein breakdown and thereby enhances the retention of protein.

5. There appears to be specific advantage to the consumption of isolated whey protein in close temporal proximity to the performance of resistance exercise. This is likely due to the high essential amino acid content as well as the rapid pattern of delivery of amino acids provided by whey.

6. Few dietary supplements have shown much advantage in promoting muscle growth aside from creation and possibly β-HMB.

Protein and increases in muscle mass

There have been a large number of nutritional compounds that have been studied as potential ergogenic (work enhancing) aids to enhance the gain in muscle mass following a period of resistance exercise training. Very few compounds have consistently been shown to have any influence whatsoever on strength or muscle mass gains following resistance exercise training. There is evidence that milk proteins are superior to soy protein with respect to protein accretion after a period of resistance exercise training and it is likely that the time course of absorption (whey = fast; casein = slow) and other bio-active components of milk protein can enhance protein retention. Recently, we noted that the effect of whey protein was superior to that of soy and casein both acutely and with chronic training studies. Thus, whey protein appears to confer some advantage over other protein sources despite quite similar amino acid profiles.

Protein timing

We now know that resistance exercise stimulates cellular events that trigger the rise in muscle protein synthesis and ultimately promote muscle growth. A number of studies have shown that it is only when protein is consumed after resistance exercise that a synergistic interaction between the exercise stimulus and the rise in amino acids that accompanies protein ingestion prompts a true net accretion of muscle protein. The result of these small periods of net muscle protein accretion can be cumulative and are what eventually sum up to become hypertrophy. The following figure summarizes data from a number of these studies. Based on these findings we recommend that protein be consumed in close temporal proximity to the performance of resistance exercise to maximize the anabolic benefits of the exercise stimulus (see figure 1 below).

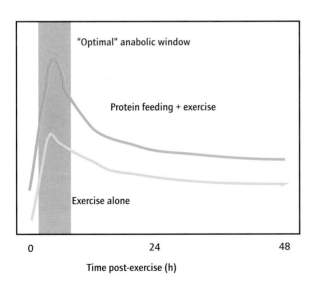

"Optimal" anabolic window

Protein feeding + exercise

Exercise alone

0   24   48

Time post-exercise (h)

Figure 1: Rate of muscle protein synthesis (MPS) after exercise with or without protein feeding. Exercise stimulates protein synthesis but it can be further increased by protein ingestion.

Schematic figure illustrating the effect of an isolated bout of resistance exercise alone on the rate of muscle protein synthesis (MPS) from rest (0h) and at 4h, 24h, and 48h post-exercise. The additive effect of feeding is shown at the same times. Note that the additive effect of feeding is greatest at 1-4h post-exercise, after ingesting protein immediately post-exercise, and diminishes with time post-exercise. Moreover, it appears that consuming milk or whey proteins at least within 1-4h after exercise is particularly advantageous in terms of promoting gains in muscle mass.

> The most effective strategy to increase strength and muscle mass is proper resistance exercise training provided adequate energy, carbohydrate and protein are consumed.

Potential ergogenic dietary supplements

There is some evidence that ,-OH-methyl butyric acid (HMB) can enhance strength gains. A recent meta-analysis of the effects of HMB (Rowlands and Thompson 2009) concluded that there were "...small but clear overall and leg strength gains in previously untrained men, but effects in trained lifters are trivial. The HMB effect on body composition is inconsequential..." Thus, to date it is hard to recommend this quite expensive supplement for resistance-trained athletes. It may be possible to make a recommendation to novice resistance-trained athletes; however, HMB has not been compared directly to an optimal nutritional regimen (early provision of carbohydrate and protein following resistance exercise training), which may ultimately be just as effective.

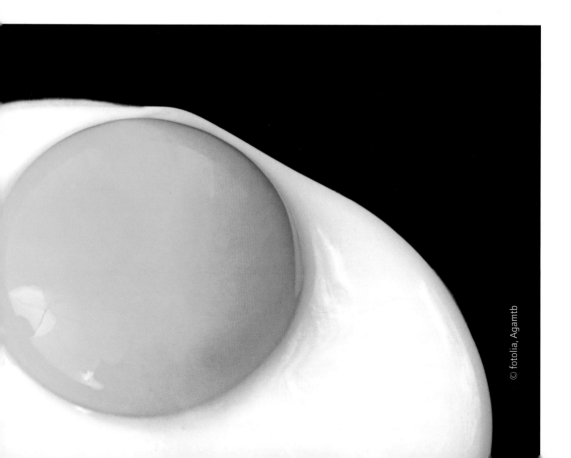

© fotolia, Agamtb

Creatine monohydrate is a guanidino compound that is synthesized in the liver, pancreas and kidney and is found in meat containing products. A number of studies have shown that creatine supplementation (5 to 10 $g^{-1} \cdot d^{-1}$) during a period of resistance exercise training can enhance the gains in fat free mass and strength. A problem with this research is that it is difficult to provide a creatine supplement in a double blind fashion and pre-existing conceptions may influence the outcome .. We have found that the early provision (within 60 min) of carbohydrate (50 g) + casein (10 g) after a work-out, given over a period of 2 months of resistance exercise training, resulted in similar strength gains when compared to training with the immediate post-exercise consumption of creatine (10 g + 50 g of carbohydrate). Based on our recent findings, we would anticipate that if whey were used, the gains in the 'control' group may have exceeded those of the creatine supplemented group.

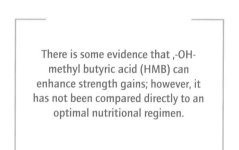

There is some evidence that ,-OH-methyl butyric acid (HMB) can enhance strength gains; however, it has not been compared directly to an optimal nutritional regimen.

The most effective strategy to increase strength and muscle mass is proper resistance exercise training with adequate energy, carbohydrate and protein consumption. A diet supplying a mixed protein source of a higher biological value (dairy, meat, eggs, isolated soy) at 1.5-1.7 $g \cdot kg^{-1} \cdot d^{-1}$ would meet the needs of essentially every athlete under any circumstance, provided that the athlete is not restricting energy intake. There does appear to be some benefit to the consumption of isolated whey proteins in the post-exercise period and reviews of training-based studies on this matter also support this contention. The timing of carbohydrate and protein replenishment in the post-exercise period is especially important to optimize protein balance and to replenish glycogen stores (particularly if an athlete is training twice a day). For a sprint/power athlete trying to put on muscle bulk and gain strength, creatine supplementation may enhance some of the strength and muscle mass gains at least during the first 4 to 6 months of training.

There is a point beyond which protein intake, whether in the form of food or protein supplements, does not make sense economically or scientifically.

Chapter 10

Train low – compete high!

Keith Baar

Glycogen loading has been known to increase endurance performance for many years (Bergstrom & Hultman 1967a). As a result, most athletes and coaches believe that training in a glycogen-loaded state is essential to optimal conditioning and performance (See also Chapter 3). However, the validity of this philosophy is now being challenged. It is becoming clear that there are benefits to training in a glycogen-depleted state. The potential benefits of training in the glycogen-depleted state have recently led many coaches and scientists to espouse a new training philosophy: "Train low-compete high". Here we will discuss the evidence in support of this philosophy as well as the potential mechanism underlying the benefits of training in a low glycogen state.

Importance of glycogen as a fuel for endurance exercise

Glycogen is the principal storage form of carbohydrate in mammals. In 1858 Claude Bernard isolated carbohydrate from liver and muscle (Bernard 1858; Young 1957). Bernard's landmark discovery provided direct evidence that muscle and liver had an accessible form of energy for meeting energy demands during exercise. Almost a century later, Bergstrom and Hultman began to investigate the role of glycogen in exercise (Bergstrom & Hultman 1966) and discovered a relationship between glycogen and exercise performance (Bergstrom et al. 1967). These early studies demonstrated that the glycogen content of a muscle is a major determinant of the capacity to sustain endurance exercise (Bergstrom & Hultman 1967a). Importantly, they also demonstrated that diet and exercise could greatly vary the glycogen content in skeletal muscle (Bergstrom et al. 1967). This final observation, that eating a high carbohydrate diet following exercise increased the recovery of muscle glycogen stores compared to a fat or protein diet, provided direct evidence that dietary glucose was the precursor for muscle glycogen (Bergstrom & Hultman 1967, 1967b) and suggested for the first time that a high muscle glycogen was beneficial for endurance performance.

Glycogen and whole body substrate utilization

In the low glycogen state, whole body metabolism shifts drastically. In humans, glycogen depletion results in increased systemic release of amino acids from muscle protein breakdown, increased fat metabolism (calculated from arterio-venous differences), reduced pyruvate oxidation, and increased levels of stress hormones such as cortisol and epinephrine (Blomstrand & Saltin 1999; Steensberg et al. 2002). As a result of these changes, it is not surprising that performance is negatively affected by low muscle glycogen. However, some have postulated that lower glycogen during training alters whole body substrate metabolism in a manner that stimulates the activation of cellular signaling pathways that might be involved in the muscular adaptation to training (Steensberg et al. 2002).

Glycogen depletion training and endurance training adaptation

In support of the beneficial effects of training in a glycogen-depleted state, Hansen et al. (2005) have shown that 10 weeks of training in a glycogen-depleted state resulted in an 85% greater increase in time to exhaustion compared with training with high glycogen. The reason for this greater increase in endurance was a larger increase in citrate synthase (CS) and 3-hydroxyacyl-CoA dehydrogenase (HAD) and other important enzymes of fat metabolism. These results have now been confirmed in highly trained cyclists suggesting that, regardless of the athlete's training state, training in a glycogen-depleted state results in an increased capacity to use fat as a fuel during exercise.

> Studies seem to suggest that regardless of how trained the athlete is, training in a glycogen-depleted state results in an increased capacity to use fat as a fuel during exercise.

Glycogen depletion training and endurance performance

Since training in the glycogen-depleted state improves the capacity for fat oxidation, this type of training might be expected to have a glycogen sparing effect during competition leading to improved performance. While this might be true for exercise at low intensities (<70% whole body VO_2max), it does not appear to have a positive effect on performance at higher intensities (>70% whole body VO_2max) where CHO are the primary fuel source. What this means is that in long duration endurance competition (triathlon, marathon, road cycling), training in a glycogen-depleted state will have a positive effect on performance. However, in shorter, higher intensity events (10K run, time trial cycling, rowing), training in a glycogen-depleted state will have less of a performance benefit. One caveat is that for competitions such as world championships and the Olympics, where heats are run prior to the finals, low glycogen training, and the resulting increase in the capacity to use fat as a fuel, may improve recovery. This, of course, is beneficial to the athlete's subsequent performance.

Resistance training it a glycogen-depleted state

In contrast to endurance training, resistance training in a glycogen-depleted state does not seem to have any beneficial effects. If anything, weight training in a glycogen-depleted state may decrease training adaptations. It is already clear that the transcriptional changes following resistance exercise are no different in a glycogen-depleted state and the greater

> For strength events, training in a glycogen-depleted state should be avoided.

metabolic stress of training with low glycogen will negatively affect the primary pathway leading to increased muscle protein synthesis. Therefore, for strength events, training in a glycogen-depleted state should be avoided.

The underlying mechanisms

Some recent work has given clues as to how training in a glycogen-depleted state results in this beneficial effect. Narkar et al. (2008) recently showed that training rats on a treadmill, while at the same time giving them a drug that activated a transcription factor called PPARẟ, resulted in the same changes that occur when training in the glycogen-depleted state: increased capacity to use fat as a fuel. Increasing the enzymes that are required for oxidizing fatty acids is what PPARẟ does. The results of this

> Exercising in the glycogen-depleted state increases circulating fatty acids and the oxidation of fat which, in turn, results in more of the byproduct that activates PPARẟ. PPARẟ is responsible for increasing the enzymes that are required for oxidizing fatty acids.

study were that the rats that trained on the treadmill and got the drug simultaneously increased their ability to run at 50% VO$_2$max by 70% over those that just ran on the treadmill. These data suggest that exercising in the glycogen-depleted state activates PPARẟ to a greater extent than training in the glycogen-loaded state. PPARẟ seems to be activated by a byproduct of the breakdown of fat in muscle. As discussed above, exercising in the glycogen-depleted state increases (the availability of) circulating fatty acids and the oxidation of fat which, in turn, results in more of the byproduct that activates PPARẟ.

How to train in a glycogen-depleted state

If you compete in long duration endurance events, or train athletes who do, a natural question is, how do I implement these techniques in my own training? The positive effects of training with low glycogen require glycogen levels to be decreased by about one third that of the normal. This can be accomplished by performing steady state exercise at 70% of max for 30 minutes to 1 hour without consuming a CHO supplement. Following the depletion stage, a second session is performed. This session can be performed immediately, or following a fast of 1-3 hours. Ideally, the second session should include high intensity work as this type of training can activate the molecular targets that improve endurance performance to their maximum (Table 1). As with all training techniques, each athlete will have to determine whether training with low glycogen affects their recovery and therefore the overall intensity of their training.

Conclusions

Training in a muscle glycogen-depleted state increases an athlete's ability to oxidize fat. In long duration endurance competition this increase in fat oxidation may spare muscle glycogen and improve performance (although performance effects are still unclear). However, in strength events and endurance events lasting less than 1 hour, where stored ATP, phosphocreatine, and CHO are the primary sources of fuel, there is no performance benefit to training in a muscle glycogen-depleted state.

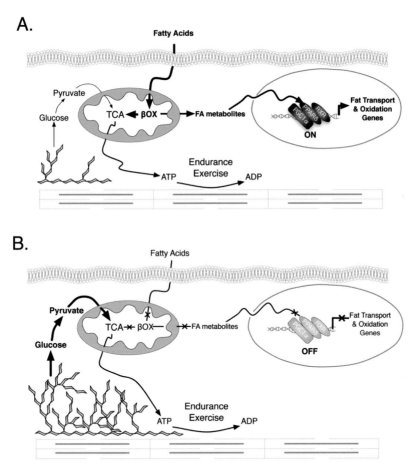

Figure 1

The potential effects of training in low muscle glycogen states on the PPAR transcription factor. A. In the low muscle glycogen state, more fatty acids are available resulting in the activation of PPARδ; B. In the high muscle glycogen state, a greater proportion of carbohydrates are used resulting in lower PPARδ activation and less adaptation of the fatty acid oxidation enzymes.

Table 1: Examples of glycogen-depletion training sessions for different sports

Sport	Depletion Session	Adaptive Session
Marathon	1h @ 75% HRmax	6 x 800m at 1 mile pace with 1.5min recovery, or 4 x 1200m at 3K race pace with 3min recovery, or 2 x 2 miles at 10K pace with 10min recovery 1h at 75% HRmax
Road Cycling	1h @ 70% HRmax	6 x 5min at 95% HRmax with 2min recovery 2 x 20min hills @ 80% Wmax
Swimming	20x 150m @ medium-high effort 15 sec rest	15 x 50m with 10sec recovery, or 10 x 200m with 20sec recovery, or 4 x 400m with 40sec recovery
	30 x 100m @ medium-high effort 15 sec rest	All with increasing intensity (1st med – last race pace)
Triathlon	4h bike with no supplementation Low CHO dinner	Morning – 3h ride with 3 x 10min @ 90% Wmax, or Morning – 1h run with 2 x 1 mile at 10K pace
Football/Soccer	30min run @75% HRmax	Regular training with team, skills sessions, repeated sprints, ball skills, etc.
Rugby/US Football, Sprinting, Rowing, Time trial cycling		This type of training is not recommended

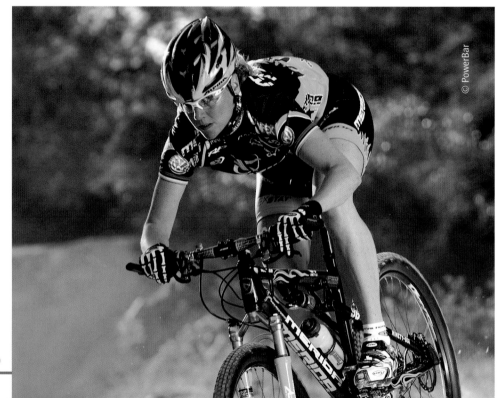

Chapter 11

Optimizing training adaptations by manipulating protein intake

Kevin Tipton

Protein is popular

The benefits of protein ingestion associated with exercise have been known for centuries. From Olympians in ancient Greece to modern Olympians in the 21st century, athletes have consumed large amounts of protein. Presently, protein supplementation is a multibillion dollar business and high protein diets are very popular with athletes. Clearly, the importance of protein nutrition is clear to athletes and other exercisers. This review will examine the impact of protein nutrition on adaptations to training. We will consider the importance of both chronic intake of protein in the diet, as well as acute supplementation of protein.

Training adaptations

The degree of adaptation to training is limited by genetics, thus top athletes can thank their parents. However, training, i.e. the type, intensity, volume, duration and other aspects of the training, have the most profound influence on protein metabolism and thus training adaptations. No matter what – or how much – is eaten, adaptations to training will be minimal without the right training stimulus and effort. Nutrition, including protein intake, may influence these adaptations to the training regimen that is practiced. It is now clear that training adaptations occur in small changes in response to each exercise bout. That means that nutrition may influence adaptations not only through overall diet throughout the training period, but also each acute response to the training session. For at least the last 20-30 years the importance of carbohydrate for optimal training has been appreciated (see also Chapters 3, 4 and 10). Other nutrients, such as fat to some extent, but in particular protein, have been receiving more attention in recent years.

Ultimately, adaptations to training result from changes in the type, quantity and activity of proteins in various tissues. For example, increased muscle mass and strength stem from increased amounts of myofibrillar, i.e. the structural, proteins in the muscle. On the other hand, increased amounts of mitochondrial proteins contribute to increased aerobic capacity with endurance training. The metabolic basis for changes in the amounts of these proteins is the balance between the rates of synthesis and breakdown of particular proteins over a given time period. For protein to be gained there must be an increase in synthesis and/or a decrease in the breakdown of that protein (see Chapter 9). Thus, the training and nutrition must influence the metabolism of proteins in various tissues for adaptations to occur.

Protein synthesis and degradation

Exercise and nutrition influence training adaptations through changes in muscle protein synthesis and breakdown that will increase (or decrease) net balance. On a daily, or even hourly, basis net balance can be either positive or negative, depending on feeding and exercise situations. The length and duration of these periods of positive and negative balance determine the net loss or gain of a protein. Consequently, in healthy, mass-stable adults, periods of positive and negative net balance will be equal, and no changes in protein content or type occur. Changes in quantity and/or type of protein only result when a cumulative positive protein net balance prevails over a period of training. Net balance of proteins changes in response to each exercise bout and associated nutritional intake. Thus, adaptations occur from the accumulation of proteins in response to each training session.

> Adaptations occur from the accumulation of proteins over time in response to each training session.

Influence of protein on protein metabolism

Protein intake may influence training adaptations in many ways. It increases muscle protein synthesis, provides amino acids for building muscle for increased muscle mass or remodeling of muscle, provides energy during exercise, and provides precursors for making hormones and other compounds important for exercise. In addition, there is mitochondrial biogenesis which is necessary for increasing muscle oxidative capacity and perhaps for glycogen re-synthesis. Thus, protein may be important both chronically and acutely.

> It is clear that the timing of protein ingestion in relation to exercise, the type of protein, the co-ingestion of other nutrients with the protein and quantity of protein ingested will all impact on the training response.

The most obvious influence of protein on changes in types or quantities of proteins with training is through its influence on protein metabolism. Exercise increases muscle protein synthesis and breakdown, but the increase in synthesis is greater than breakdown. Thus, the response of net muscle protein balance, i.e. the metabolic basis for changes in proteins that result in adaptations, is an increase. However, without a source of amino acids, such as amino acid or protein supplements or protein in foods, the balance remains negative, i.e. there is no net gain of protein. Ingestion of protein following exercise, whether resistance or endurance exercise, results in increased muscle protein synthesis and positive net muscle protein balance. Thus, it is clear that protein ingestion with exercise will influence training adaptations. Unfortunately, the optimal amount or type of protein to ingest to maximize training adaptations is still unknown. At this point, we do know that factors, such as the timing of protein ingestion in relation to exercise, the type of protein, coingestion of other nutrients with the protein and quantity of protein ingested, will impact the response. Moreover, the type of exercise, intensity of exercise, volume of the training bout and other factors influence the response of muscle protein metabolism. When you consider how many interactions of these variables there may be, it should be clear that determination of the optimal response is very complex and we have a long way to go before we know the best combination of these factors for various desired adaptations to exercise. Nonetheless, over the past 15, and especially the last 5, years, researchers have made strides toward better understanding of the response. In this chapter, we will offer insights into the current state of affairs with regard to protein nutrition and training adaptations.

Timing of protein ingestion in relation to exercise

There has been a great deal of attention on the importance of timing of protein ingestion in recent years. It is amply clear that the response of muscle protein metabolism differs depending on when the protein is ingested in relation to exercise. In fact, many believe that protein must be ingested in close temporal proximity to exercise to optimize the response. In fact, many articles and books claim that protein must be ingested within as little as 45 min after exercise to reap the benefits – the so called "metabolic window". Whereas there is some support for the general notion that protein should be ingested in close proximity to the exercise (see Chapter 9), the evidence suggests that the story is more complex than that.

Acute studies suggest that the response of muscle anabolism is maximized at different times depending on what type of amino acid source is consumed and whether or not other nutrients are ingested along with protein. It is clear that ingestion of protein immediately prior to exercise engenders an anabolic response similar to that of the response seen when it is ingested after exercise. Thus, the 45 min post exercise window must be expanded to include at least a few minutes prior to exercise. Furthermore, there is recent evidence that the response of muscle protein synthesis to exercise is similar when a protein-containing meal is consumed 1.5h prior to exercise and protein or amino acids are ingested following exercise. Finally, given that the response of muscle protein synthesis to exercise lasts for up to 48-72 h after the exercise, it, again, does not seem warranted to limit the interactive effect to the first 45 min only. In fact, a recent study presented at a scientific conference demonstrated that there was an interactive effect of protein consumption 24h after exercise. Clearly, evidence suggests that the "metabolic window" for the effectiveness of protein intake should not be limited to only a short time after exercise.

As usual, the timing story is more complex than we would like. However, there does not seem to be any reason that an athlete should not consume some protein immediately after exercise. At this point, we don't know if the response immediately after exercise is greater than that at 24h post exercise. If so, there may be some small, yet important, advantage to eating protein immediately after exercise. It certainly does not seem possible that it could be detrimental, as long as the protein fits into the total energy budget. Thus, taking a cost-benefit approach, it is still advisable to eat protein after exercise even if the evidence for the benefits may have been a bit overstated.

Type of amino acid source and other nutrients

The response of muscle protein metabolism following exercise varies depending on the source of amino acids ingested and whether or not other nutrients are ingested. As with the timing issue, there is no definitive recommendation that can be made at present. However, there are a few recent observations that are interesting and may help us to formulate some kind of advice (see also Chapter 9). It seems that animal proteins may provide a superior response in muscle. The digestive properties of the protein may be important in this regard. As such, there is recent evidence that whey protein ingestion following resistance exercise results in a superior response of muscle protein synthesis compared to casein and soy protein (as discussed in Chapter 9). However, another study showed that there was no difference in the anabolic response of net muscle protein balance between whey protein and casein ingestion following exercise. The difference between the studies may be due to differences in the response of muscle protein breakdown. Thus, the bottom line anabolic response is no different. Given that exercise intensity also seems to impact the anabolic response – and there is no information on the interaction of intensity and type of protein – the specific type of protein to ingest in any given situation cannot be recommended.

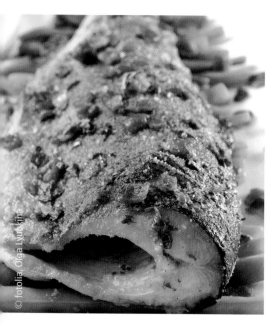

© fotolia, Olga Lyubkina

In addition to the type of protein, there is evidence that the anabolic response following exercise may be influenced by other nutrients ingested with the protein. That means that the response to protein ingestion after exercise will be different if carbohydrates, fats or both are ingested along with the protein. Many recommendations ignore this aspect of the nutritional influence on the anabolic response to exercise. Again, this factor should be considered when particular recommendations are made.

Finally, given that the training status of the individual influences the response of muscle protein metabolism to exercise, it follows that this factor also should be investigated with regard to how protein will be utilized. However, to date, there are no studies specifically investigating this aspect of adaptations to training. Obviously, there is much more to be learned before we can determine what is the best.

Amount of protein

The ideal amount of protein to ingest following exercise is considered the Holy Grail by many. Some, especially strength athletes, try to consume as much protein as possible after exercise. However, this approach may not be optimal. There is now evidence that ingestion of excess protein – above that which can be synthesized into proteins in muscle – is simply de-animated and oxidized for energy. A recent study suggests that anything above 20-25 g of protein is excess and could be considered a waste. As usual, there are many questions to be answered before an absolute amount can be recommended. How does the type of exercise, the intensity of exercise, the type of protein and other aforementioned aspects of exercise training and nutrition influence this relationship? At this point, given the information available, there is no reason to recommend more than 20-25 g of protein following exercise.

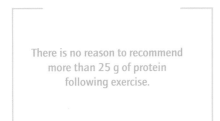

There is no reason to recommend more than 25 g of protein following exercise.

Importance of supplemental protein

There are many advocates of the superiority of supplemental protein sources. They believe protein supplements are superior to food sources of protein. However, there is no evidence that food sources of protein result in metabolic responses or training adaptations inferior to those from protein in supplement form. In fact, there is ample evidence that the response of muscle metabolism is similar. On the other hand, it may be difficult for many athletes to consume a meal and a protein supplement may be a valuable asset in their nutritional regimen. Given the busy training schedules, convenience is an aspect of any training/nutrition regimen that should not be overlooked when making recommendations to athletes.

Total dietary protein

Many scientists believe that the amount of protein that athletes need to consume is more than sedentary individuals, but the exact amount is highly individual and dependent on many factors. Moreover, the amount of protein ingested is less important than other factors, such as the ones we mentioned previously. Nevertheless, athletic governing bodies and scientific organizations have attempted to define the optimal protein intake for (strength and endurance) athletes. Typically, the recommendation for strength athletes is 1.4-1.7 g protein$\cdot$kg$^{-1}\cdot$d^{-1} body mass/day or somewhere in that range. For endurance athletes the recommendations tend to be slightly lower – usually around 1.2-1.6 g protein$\cdot$kg$^{-1}\cdot$d^{-1} body mass$\cdot$day. These estimates are based primarily on studies that utilize nitrogen balance (NBAL) methodology. Whereas, these studies were performed by excellent researchers, as meticulously as possible, interpretation of the data from studies using the NBAL technique is fraught with peril.

The recommendations for protein intake must be considered very loosely and should be taken as a starting point. Clearly, there are many types of athletes who do not fall neatly into the two broad categories of strength or endurance. Some wouldn't be considered either of these and others would be considered both. They, too, would welcome such recommendations. Furthermore, there are many dietary factors, in addition to the quantity of protein, which impact training adaptations to training. The type of protein or amino acid source, the timing of intake in relation to exercise, co-ingestion of other nutrients with protein, all influence the response of muscle. Two identical athletes eating the same amount of protein may experience different adaptations depending on these and other factors. Therefore, the exact recommendation for protein for any athlete should be based on the particular situation for that athlete. Specifically, total energy intake, carbohydrate and fat needs, pattern of protein intake, as well as training characteristics should all be taken into account. Reliance only on broad recommendations must be considered a mistake.

> Whereas for a reasonably high protein intake may not be harmful, there is currently no evidence that protein intake above 1.5 to maybe 2.0 g·kg^{-1}·d^{-1} is beneficial.

Many athletes feel that a high protein intake (above 2.0 g·kg^{-1}·d^{-1} up to 3-4 g·kg^{-1}·d^{-1}) is necessary for optimal adaptation, especially for increased mass and strength. However, as long ago as 1907 up to very recently, studies have clearly demonstrated that muscle mass can be gained on a wide variety of protein intakes as long as other dietary factors are not compromised. Again, although high protein intakes may not be harmful to some, there is currently no evidence that protein intake above 1.5 to maybe 2.0 g protein·kg^{-1}·d^{-1} is beneficial. Given the relatively high energy intakes necessary to support training, most athletes will easily get enough protein in a normal diet. However, it should be noted that for some, perhaps smaller athletes with lower energy intakes, more consideration needs to be given to assure appropriate protein intakes.

Risks of extra protein

Any discussion of a high protein diet for athletes should include the risks of excessive protein consumption. There has been much written about the dangers to bone and kidneys if protein intake is consistently high. However, there is no evidence that kidney problems will develop, in otherwise healthy individuals, on the basis of protein intake. If, however, an athlete has an underlying kidney problem, then a high protein intake could be problematic and even dangerous. As for bone, as long as the diet includes sufficient fruits and vegetables, potential acidosis from a high protein diet should not cause any loss of calcium from bone. Furthermore, it should be remembered that bone is not all calcium. The matrix of bone is collagen – a protein that responds well to protein intake. Thus, there is an argument that bone health could be improved by proper protein intake. The major problem with excess protein intake for athletes is that it usually comes at the expense of other nutrients given the limit on energy which one can consume. Most often protein replaces carbohydrate (and sometimes fat) which are crucial for proper training. In this way, excess protein intake could impair the ability to train at appropriate levels due to lack of necessary nutrients. The operative factor is that each athlete, coach and/or nutrition advisor

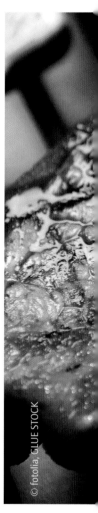

© fotolia, GLUE STOCK

should carefully consider the individual needs of the athlete and not rely on general recommendations for protein – or for that matter, any other nutrient.

Given the myriad of interactions to consider when thinking of the influence of protein on adaptations to training, it may seem that no recommendations are possible. There is no way to generalize the optimal amount, type, timing, or combinations of nutrients ingested for all exercise types including the two general types that are commonly considered. However, given the aforementioned cost-benefit approach and some generalizations, it should be possible to make some practical recommendations. For example, since animal proteins seem superior and there is the suggestion that ingesting protein soon after exercise may be helpful, why not recommend a high quality, animal protein after exercise. Most likely, the athlete will be eating soon after the exercise and the meal will include protein. However, if not, a protein supplement could be recommended. The key is that an individual approach should be adopted based on all available information related to factors that may improve or impair the training of that athlete.

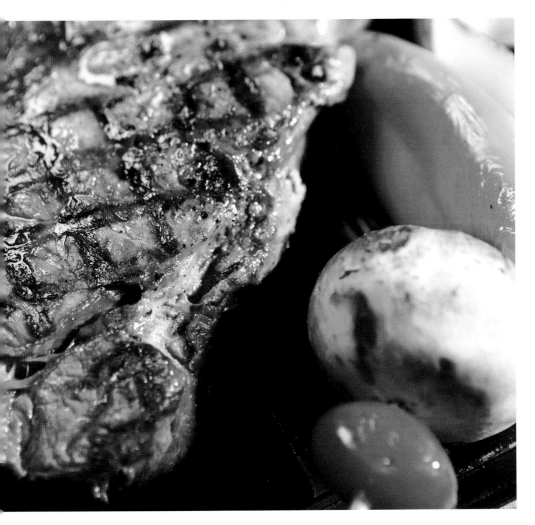

The myth	The evidence
Large amounts of protein are required to increase muscle mass.	Increased mass and strength are possible on a wide range of protein intakes as long as energy balance is maintained. There is no scientific evidence that excessive amounts (>1.7- 2.0g protein·kg body mass·d) are necessary for gains in muscle mass. Excess protein is oxidized, rather than utilized for muscle building.
Protein requirements for endurance and strength trained athletes have been determined.	There is disagreement among scientists about the requirements for protein intake for athletes. Requirements refer to the minimal amount necessary to function. Obviously, athletes and coaches are not concerned merely with requirements, but should focus on recommendations.
Recommended protein intakes for athletes should be based on protein requirements for optimal training adaptations.	Protein intake should be individually determined for each athlete based on many factors. For example, training status and type, intensity and duration of training, energy requirements and requirements for other nutrients, as well as other factors such as age, gender and injury status should all be considered.
Whey protein is the best type of protein.	There is insufficient evidence to conclude that any particular type of protein is superior to all others.
Protein supplements are the best way to increase protein intake.	There is no evidence to suggest that protein in supplement form is superior to protein ingested as part of foods. Recent research demonstrates that food protein results in muscle anabolic responses similar to that from protein supplements or free amino acids.
The total amount of protein is the most important consideration for optimal training adaptations.	Given a minimal amount of protein intake, approximately 1-1.2g protein·kg^{-1}·d^{-1}, other factors associated with protein ingestion (timing of protein intake in relation to exercise, type of protein, other nutrients ingested with the protein) and their interaction must be considered. These factors will all contribute to the response of muscle.
Many athletes need to increase their protein intake.	Studies show that the vast majority of athletes eat ample protein in their normal diet. Increased protein intake is unnecessary for most. Individual assessments should be made of each athlete's diet to determine if more protein is necessary before a concerted effort to increase intake is made.

Strategies for protein consumption	The evidence
When	Protein ingestion in close proximity – shortly before and/or within 2h following - to exercise may provide the optimal conditions to maximize training adaptations, especially for increased muscle mass and strength. However, recent evidence suggests that the necessity for this tactic has been overstated. A normal dietary pattern of protein intake will support adaptations to training.
What	There is mounting evidence that the type of protein ingested may influence training adaptations. For example, recent studies indicate that ingestion of animal proteins will result in superior gains in mass and strength over plant sources. Essential amino acids in free form may also offer some advantages, but the impact for athletes is unclear.
How	Protein is found in many food sources, such as meats, fish, egg, dairy, legumes (beans and peas) and other vegetables. There is no evidence to suggest that protein supplements provide superior adaptations over food sources. There is evidence that consumption of protein with carbohydrates and, possibly, fats may influence adaptations, particularly in terms of gains in muscle mass.
How much	Many scientists, coaches and athletes believe that athletes need to ingest more protein than non active individuals. However, there is no evidence to support the necessity or even benefit for very high protein intakes, i.e. >1.7-2.0 g protein·kg bw·day. Given the high energy intakes of most athletes, protein intake is likely adequate without supplements or additional effort. Excess protein intake may impair training adaptations if consumed at the expense of other nutrients, particularly carbohydrates that are necessary to support training.

Chapter 12

Alternative fuels

Asker Jeukendrup

Alternative fuels, also known as non-conventional fuels, are any materials or substances that can be used as a fuel other than conventional fuels. The conventional fuels for the athlete are fatty acids and glucose. Because a larger CO_2 production would generally be indicative of better performance in athletes, we may be looking for ways to increase their carbon footprint rather than reducing it. Nevertheless, the search for alternative fuels continues.

Carbohydrate and fat are the most important fuels for the human body. Both fuels are stored in the body: the carbohydrate stores are small and can be exhausted within a couple of hours, the fat stores are virtually unlimited but it is difficult to tap into this source of fuel at high exercise intensities. Making sure the fuel tank is full with carbohydrate at the start of exercise has been shown to improve endurance capacity and topping it up by consuming carbohydrate during exercise can further enhance performance. However it is also known that glucose when

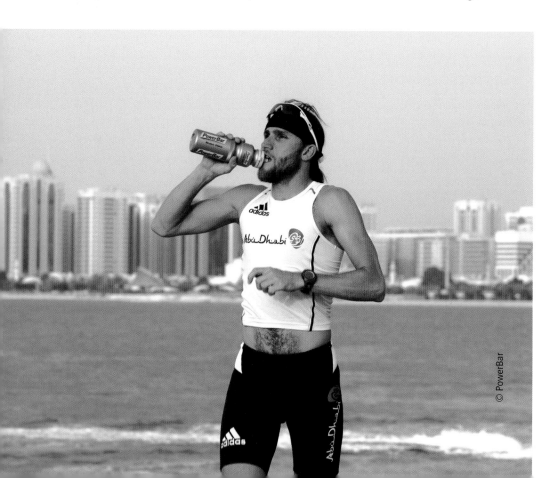

© PowerBar

ingested during exercise cannot be oxidized at rates much higher than 60 grams or 240 kcal per hour. With carbohydrate oxidation rates usually well above 500 kcal per hour during moderate intensity exercise for a moderately to well trained trained person and around 1000 kcal per hour for top athletes, the body's carbohydrate stores will still be reduced very rapidly. Therefore, the search for alternative or additional fuels for athletes has continued. Table 1 summarizes the evidence regarding a number of alternative fuels.

Different types of carbohydrates

Initially we experimented with different types of carbohydrate to see if any of them could be metabolized faster than glucose. We studied galactose, maltose, sucrose, maltodextrins, and different types of starches. We found that some of these carbohydrates were oxidized just as fast as glucose; the oxidation never exceeded 60 grams per hour. More recently we studied two relatively new carbohydrates: trehalose and isomaltulose but we found that these carbohydrates were oxidized 50-60% slower than maltose. We also studied a very high molecular weight glucose polymer (HMW-GP) a very large starch molecule) (Rowland et al. 2005). Previously such a HMW-GP had been shown to enhance gastric emptying compared with glucose. Another advantage of this HMW-GP would be that the osmolality is low, even at high concentrations of carbohydrate. However, oxidation rates were comparable to glucose (Rowland et al. 2005). In conclusion, no single carbohydrate can outperform glucose in terms of oxidation (Jeukendrup 2008).

Combinations of carbohydrates

After discoveringthat the most likely reason for a ceiling of about 60 gram per hour in oxidation rates of ingested carbohydrate was because of a limitation on absorption, we started to experiment with different types of carbohydrate. The theory was that if carbohydrate transporters in the intestine become saturated, no further oxidation can occur. This would mean that ingesting more of the same carbohydrate would have no effect on the oxidation of ingested carbohydrate. We hypothesized that by introducing a different carbohydrate, which uses a different transporter, that carbohydrate would be oxidized as well and increase the overall rate of exogenous carbohydrate (ingested carbohydrate) oxidation. This proved successful as the ingestion of combinations of glucose and fructose, maltodextrins and fructose and glucose and sucrose all resulted in higher oxidation rates (Jeukendrup and Mosely 2008). In two studies oxidation rates were around 110 grams per hour (Jentjens and Jeukendrup 2005).

In all these studies a few observations were made that are important from a practical point of view. First, there is no magical optimal ratio of glucose and fructose. Secondly, fructose is often associated with gastrointestinal distress but when ingested with glucose these problems seem to disappear. Thirdly, in order to see a positive effect on oxidation and performance, relatively large amounts of carbohydrate have to be ingested. However when ingested at rates of 90 g·h glucose:fructose drinks do work and can substantially improve performance compared with a carbohydrate drink with only one type of carbohydrate (Currell and Jeukendrup 2008).

Table 1: Examples of alternative fuels and the evidence to support their use

Alternative fuel	Evidence	Recommended
Galactose	Oxidized at lower rates than glucose	No
Isomaltulose	Oxidized at lower rates than glucose	No
Trehalose	Oxidized at lower rates than glucose	No
Maltodextrins	Oxidized at rates similar to glucose and less sweet	*
Heavy molecular weight glucose polymers	Oxidized at rates similar to glucose, less sweet but difficult to dissolve in water	*
Multiple transportable carbohydrates (i.e. glucose plus fructose; maltodextrins plus fructose)	Oxidized at higher rates than glucose only, better water delivery, improved performance, good tolerance	***
Carbohydrate plus protein	Mixed results, insufficient evidence to support its use	No
BCAA	Unlikely to be an important fuel, no effects shown on performance	No
MCT	Oxidized rapidly but causes GI distress	No
Lactate salts	Causes GI distress in larger amounts	No
Poly lactate	Poor bioavailability, can cause GI discomfort and no shown effects	No

Caffeine and glucose

When you add a fuel additive to the fuel in your car you can save money while increasing fuel efficiency and lubricity and reducing fuel emissions. Caffeine may have a similar role when ingested with carbohydrate. It has been shown that caffeine co-ingested with carbohydrate resulted in 26% higher exogenous carbohydrate oxidation rates, presumably by improving the absorption of glucose. In this study the amount of caffeine was relatively large and the amount of carbohydrate relatively low. In a follow up study with lower doses of carbohydrate we showed that exogenous carbohydrate oxidation was not increased. However caffeine has been shown to enhance performance independent of an effect on exogenous carbohydrate oxidation (see Chapter 18). More research needs to be done in order to determine in what conditions caffeine can be a useful fuel additive.

Medium Chain Triglyceride (MCT)

Because we initially believed that carbohydrate could not be oxidized at rates higher than 60 grams per hour, we started to look into fuels that were not carbohydrate but could provide energy quickly. One such fuel was MCT. MCTs are relatively small fats that empty from the stomach rapidly, are rapidly absorbed and can also be oxidized rapidly. In a first series of studies we added MCT to a carbohydrate drink and confirmed that MCT was oxidized rapidly and completely. However, because we only gave relative small amounts (30 grams over the course of 3 hours) no changes were seen in metabolism or performance. It was difficult to give larger amounts of MCT as this typically produced lower abdominal problems. When athletes adapted to a high MCT intake, there was an attenuation of the gastro-intestinal distress, there were some adaptations in metabolism but repeated sprint performance was actually decreased.

Branched chain amino acid (BCAA) ingestion during exercise

It has been suggested that branched chain amino acids (BCAA) can act as a fuel during exercise, in addition to carbohydrate and fat. However, the activities of the enzymes involved in the oxidation of BCAAs were shown to be too low to allow a major contribution of BCAAs to energy expenditure. Detailed studies with a labeled BCAA showed that the oxidation of BCAAs only increases 2-fold to 3-fold during exercise, whereas the oxidation of carbohydrate and fat increases 10-fold to 20-fold.

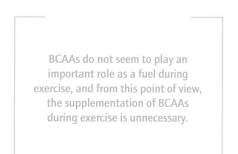

BCAAs do not seem to play an important role as a fuel during exercise, and from this point of view, the supplementation of BCAAs during exercise is unnecessary.

Also, carbohydrate ingestion during exercise can prevent the increase in BCAA oxidation. A related claim is that BCAAs can spare glycogen because they are used as a fuel instead of muscle glycogen. Studies, however, have clearly not found this to be the case during exercise with BCAA ingestion. In three very well-controlled studies no effects of BCAA supplementation on performance were seen. Using a time trial and exercise to voluntary exhaustion, these studies found no effect of BCAA ingestion on performance. BCAAs, therefore, do not seem to play an important role as a fuel during exercise, and from this point of view, the supplementation of BCAAs during exercise is unnecessary.

Protein ingestion during exercise

Recently there has been a lot of discussion about a possible role for protein during exercise. The excitement of protein added to carbohydrate drinks stems from a small number of studies that suggested that adding a small amount of protein (2% whey protein or about 20 grams per liter) to a carbohydrate drink produced improvements in endurance capacity compared to a sports drink alone. These studies have been criticized for various reasons. The subjects used in these studies were not trained, the diet in the days leading up to the experiment was not carefully controlled and there were (technical) problems in the way the exercise performance tests were conducted.

Exercise scientists were baffled by these findings when they were published because it is difficult to think of a mechanism by which protein would have such effects! Interestingly, the same authors repeated their study a couple of years later and did not find an effect on performance. In several recent, very well-controlled studies a carbohydrate + protein beverage provided no additional performance benefit.

> Although there are some suggestions that protein can have an additive performance effect to carbohydrate when ingested during prolonged exercise, well-controlled studies do not seem to confirm this. Therefore, at present, there is not enough evidence to recommend protein during exercise.

Lactate salts and polylactate

Lactate is a good fuel for the human heart and muscle, and the rate of lactate clearance and oxidation in several studies exceeded those rates achieved by glucose. Most of the lactate that appears in the blood during moderate-intensity exercise is oxidized by the active muscle fibers with a high oxidative capacity. Lactate can be provided as sodium or potassium lactate. However, a solution containing these salts has a very high osmolarity. The amounts of sodium or potassium that would have to be ingested are very large and are likely to produce severe gastro-intestinal problems. Solutions of lactate salts can be taken in maximal bolus amounts of about 10 g without causing gastro-intestinal problems.

Theoretically this problem of too much lactate salt could be solved by using polylactate, a lactate polymer, which would reduce the osmolarity yet provide relatively large amounts of lactate. Polylactate is used as a supplement and is included in some sports drinks. If polylactate dissolved better in water and could be quickly hydrolyzed in the gastro-intestinal tract of humans, like glucose polymers, it could be the ideal chemical form in which to ingest carbohydrate. However, polylactate does not normally occur in food products and does not

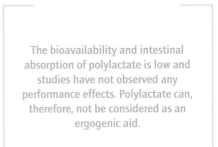

> The bioavailability and intestinal absorption of polylactate is low and studies have not observed any performance effects. Polylactate can, therefore, not be considered as an ergogenic aid.

dissolve very well in water. In addition, the human body does not contain enzymes to degrade polylactate. Thus, the bioavailability and intestinal absorption are very low or even zero. In the true chemical sense, polylactate cannot generate lactate at a high rate, or function as a nutritional ergogenic aid during exercise. Studies have also not observed any performance effects. Polylactate can, therefore, not be considered as an ergogenic aid. The main problem with lactate supplements (in each of the available forms) is that performance effects can only be expected at ingestion rates that are not tolerated by the gastro-intestinal tract.

Conclusions

- Certain carbohydrate blends (such as glucose and fructose) can improve delivery of carbohydrate and fluid compared with single carbohydrates. This has also been shown to improve performance. However, in order to be effective large amounts of carbohydrate have to be ingested (>90 g·h⁻¹).
- Caffeine is a stimulant and can improve endurance performance. A low dose (2-3 mg·kg⁻¹) will already have this effect. Larger doses do not provide additional benefit.
- Some studies have suggested that consuming protein with CHO during exercise improves endurance capacity (time to exhaustion) while other studies have reported no benefits. Additional research will resolve this debate, but it should be remembered that there is no established mechanism by which protein intake during exercise should improve performance.
- BCAA do not seem to contribute much as a fuel and do not improve endurance performance.
- Lactate and polylactate are interesting alternative fuels but in the amounts found in products they do not add much as a fuel.
- MCTs are an interesting fuel but when ingested in large quantities causes gastrointestinal distress and in smaller amounts (<30g) have no effect.

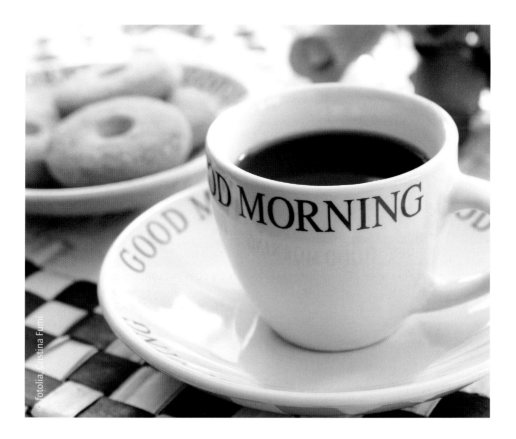

© Fotolia_Cristina Fumi

Chapter 13

Dietary Supplements

Hans Braun

The term "dietary supplement" implies that this is something that supplements the normal diet. Indeed leading sport organizations recommend that "athletes should ensure they have a good diet before contemplating supplement use" (Maughan et al. 2007). It is interesting to note that recent reports show that only 54 % (Olympic athletes) and 18 % (elite young athletes) have had experience with individual nutritional consulting (Braun et al. 2009) and, therefore, their knowledge about what an optimal normal diet is may be somewhat limited. On the other hand, many studies have demonstrated that the use of dietary supplements is widespread (76 % - 91 %) among athletes (Braun et al. 2009; Maughan et al. 2007) although these data may be influenced by what products are classified as dietary supplement.

> The use of dietary supplements is widespread among athletes.

The term "dietary supplement" is not used consistently in the scientific literature and no clear definition is available for supplements which are explicitly used by athletes (Maughan et al. 2007). Athletes use a wide variety of products that could be classified as dietary supplement: sports drinks, carbohydrate-rich energy products, protein and protein components, vitamins, minerals, trace elements, herbal extracts and ergogenic aids (caffeine, buffering agents, and creatine). Athletes use supplements for different reasons but the main motives for using supplements are usually optimizing regeneration and immune function, improving general health and increasing performance.

> The term "dietary supplement" is not used consistently in the scientific literature and no clear definition is available for supplements which are explicitly used by athletes.

The benefit of most dietary supplements is still under debate because their effectiveness is often not scientifically proven. Reasons for that might be: individual differences in response and tolerance, the placebo effect of taking supplement or simply the lack of research. It is important to consider the available evidence before deciding to advise or use a dietary supplement. Both the risks and benefits of dietary supplements need to be discussed before turning to a supplement. Recent studies show that physicians, coaches, nutritionists, physiotherapists and parents are the main providers of information about dietary supplements (Braun et al. 2007). Therefore, not only athletes need to be educated about the use of supplements.

Sports drinks – carbohydrate-rich solutions

Sports drinks are designed to rapidly deliver fluid and fuel during and after exercise. Several recommendations are available on the optimal composition of a sports drink. In general, a sports drink during exercise should contain carbohydrates (6-8 %), sodium (20-30 mmol·L^{-1} and potassium (3-5 mmol·L^{-1}) (ACSM, 2007). However the mixture depends on climate situation (cold or hot environment), the carbohydrate or fluid needs (dilution of the drink) and individual tolerance (see also Chapters 4, 5 and 25).

The use of sports drinks might be beneficial to performance of high intensity exercise, endurance events, prolonged intermittent exercise (team sports) or in weight class sports for quick recovery after weigh-in. Sports drinks are designed for active people during exercise and recovery and their effectiveness depends on the duration and also the intensity of exercise. One should question whether those who spend a few minutes in the gym each day, often with the goal to lose weight, should be encouraged to consume carbohydrate containing beverages.

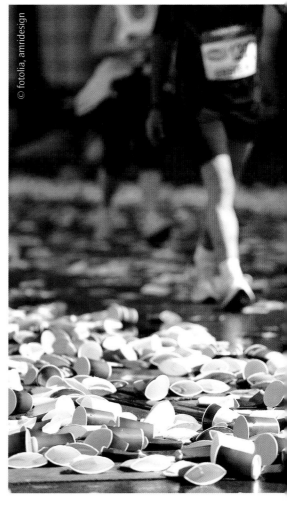

Sport gels and sport bars – carbohydrate-rich sport food

A carbohydrate replacement during exercise might be beneficial for high intensity exercise of > 1 hour (Jeukendrup 2008). Sports gels and bars are compact and portable sources of carbohydrates. They provide a relatively large fuel boost in a single serving. To meet hydration needs and to reduce the risk of gastrointestinal intolerance they should be consumed with adequate fluid.

Carbohydrate-rich supplements are not only beneficial during intensive exercise; they also provide compact energy for quick recovery when hunger is suppressed, when solid food is not available or as a snack between two training sessions. However, these supplements should only be used under specific conditions for which they are suited rather than as a general snack. Gels and bars are very energy dense and, if overused, can lead to a high energy intake or an inappropriate replacement of whole foods. Therefore, food sources should always be considered as the first option for meals and snacks.

Protein and protein components

The recommendations for protein intake in athletes are described with a maximum requirement of approximately 1.7 g per kg body mass (Tranopolsky 2008). Dietary surveys show that the dietary patterns of athletes provide protein intakes of 1.2-2.0 $g \cdot kg^{-1}$ BM per day as long as energy requirements are met. However if, a higher protein intake for athletes is necessary, it can be met with protein-rich food sources s (e.g. dairy products, meat, fish, cereals, soy, some vegetables). Given the wide range of food choices, protein supplements are not necessary.

> There is little evidence to support a benefit of amino acid supplementation for athletes with a normal diet.

With regard to the timing of protein intake, it has been suggested that protein intake should take place immediately following exercise. However, recent reviews discussing this aspect conclude that it still seems unclear if there is a real benefit for athletes following this strategy (Hawley et al. 2007; Tipton 2008).

A protein-carbohydrate snack or meal after a strenuous workout seems to be a possible choice for muscle repair, adaptation to training and to provide carbohydrate fuel to restore muscle glycogen levels (Tarnopolsky 2008). However, this does not necessarily have to be juin the form of a carbohydrate-protein bar, drink or powder, as the same nutrients can be provided by a food based snack or meal (see Chapter 11). In the case of amino acids, there is little evidence to support a benefit of supplementation for athletes with a normal diet (Maughan et al. 2007).

Vitamins, minerals and trace elements

While Recommended Dietary Allowances (RDA) are guidelines for the intake of vitamins, minerals and trace elements for the general population, official recommendations for athletes do not exist. Over the years, even conferences on sports nutrition have not been able to reach a consensus about the additional micronutrient needs for athletes. In contrast, an earlier report stated that: "scientific evidence is lacking or inconsistent in supporting recommendations for nutritional intakes beyond the accepted dietary guidelines." (European Commission 2009) Even if single studies might support a higher intake of micronutrients it seems that much more research is needed in this field to get a clear statement.

Athletes often take single nutrients (iron, magnesium, vitamin C, vitamin E, etc.) without any knowledge of their dietary or biochemical status. They should be aware that an over-supplementation could cause negative effects on health and performance (European Food Safety Authority 2009). Therefore, supplements (e.g. iron) should be taken under medical supervision and after nutritional assessment by a sports dietitian.

It is generally accepted that athletes need an adequate intake of all micronutrients and their needs seem to be higher compared to the sedentary population. However, these nutrients are best obtained from a varied diet based largely on nutrient-rich food. In a period of restricted energy intake, athletes may be at risk of inadequate nutrient intake. Furthermore, when food intake cannot be balanced (athletes traveling in countries with limited food supply) or food choices cannot be improved, a multi-vitamin-mineral supplement might be helpful.

Upper intake levels of vitamins and minerals

In addition to the supplementation of nutrients, the fortification of foods has become very popular during the past years. In supermarkets, Many foods enriched with micronutrients can be found in supermarkets, such as yoghurts, juice, sweets and many sports food items, to name a few. Sports drinks or bars, for example, which are mainly intended for carbohydrate delivery, contain a package of micronutrients although a scientific reason for this is not given. However, can this be harmful? The European Food Safety Authority (2009) established tolerable intake levels for vitamins and minerals (UL). The UL is defined as the "maximum level of total chronic daily intake of a nutrient (from all sources) judged to be unlikely to pose a risk of adverse health effects to humans." (European Food Safety Authority, 2009) For example, the UL for magnesium (only supplementation) is established at 250 mg per day, while for zinc a UL of daily total intake (food + supplementation) lies in a range of 25 mg for adults and 18-22 mg for adolescents. These dosages can easily be taken by supplements or by the combination of sports food (sports drink + sports bar + multi-vitamin-mineral supplement) enriched with micronutrients.

In sum, even if it is unclear what doses are harmful for athletes, vitamins and minerals should be accounted for in the supplementation strategy and the choice of sports food.

Ergogenic aids and other substances

Many products claiming to increase performance, health status or improved regeneration are offered on the supplement market. Yet, there is good evidence on efficiency and safety for only a few substances. The absence of evidence does not mean a product is ineffective or that it is without risk for health or decreased performance (Maughan et al. 2007).

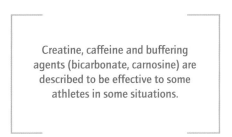

Creatine, caffeine and buffering agents (bicarbonate, carnosine) are described to be effective to some athletes in some situations.

Furthermore, if evidence exists, it does not mean that this works in all athletes in all situations. Supplement use requires individual assessment based on type of sport, nutritional status, training status and genotype. Therefore, athletes need to find out if they respond positively to the use of a supplement. They should be aware about dosage, time (e.g. before, after exercise) and period of using the supplement. Creatine, caffeine and buffering agents (bicarbonate, carnosine) are described to be effective to some athletes in some situations (Maughan et al. 2007).

Risk – contamination and doping

Since 1999 the risk of dietary supplements being contaminated with doping substances has been well described (Geyer 2008). These studies showed that supplements may contain prohibited substances. An international study performed in 2001/2002 on 634 supplements showed about 15% of non-hormonal supplements to be contaminated with anabolic-androgenic steroids. In 2005 vitamin C, multivitamin and magnesium tablets were confiscated, which contained cross contaminations of stanozolol and metandienone. Furthermore, some dietary supplements have been found to contain high amounts of anabolic steroids (Geyer 2008). This will be discussed further in Chapter 14. Experts in the field expect that the contamination of dietary supplements on the market will get worse in the future, due to an increased trade and availability of anabolic steroids, especially from China (Geyer 2008). Therefore, athletes are advised to take supplements only from "low-risk" sources. Databases in Germany (www.colognelist.com) and the Netherlands (http://antidoping.nl/nzvt) list supplements from companies with high quality control standards, which screen for anabolic steroids and stimulants and guarantee that the products have had no contact with these substances in the production and transportation processes.

Table 1: Risks and benefits of dietary supplements

	Benefit	Risk
In general	psychological aid / placebo effect	inadvertent doping cases and health risk
Sports drinks	delivers fluid and carbohydrates during exercise post exercise rehydration and refueling	high energy density nutrient density low
Carbohydrate-rich products	training periods with high carbohydrate needs carbo-loading before competition during and after exercise for refueling	high energy density nutrient density low
Protein	to meet protein needs in periods with low caloric intake	
Vitamins, Minerals, Trace Elements	during restricted energy intake in periods of an unbalanced diet (e.g. travelling, busy schedule) to meet daily micronutrient recommendations	be aware of intakes higher than upper intake levels
Ergogenic Aids	for some athletes in some circumstances creatine, caffeine, buffering agents might be of benefit	side effects are possible, check individual response

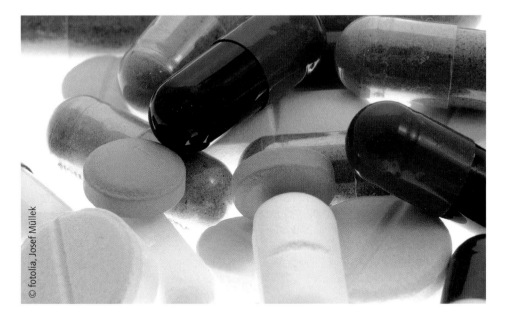

© fotolia, Josef Müllek

Conclusions

Before contemplating supplement use:
* Athletes should ensure having a healthy, balanced and sport specific diet.
* For implementation, individual nutritional assessment by a qualified sports nutrition professional is advised.
* The intake of micronutrients coming from fortified (sports) food should not be underestimated and can lead to an intake higher than the upper intake level.
* Supplements can be contaminated or faked with illegal substances and can lead to a positive doping case.

Dietary supplements cannot simply be classified into the categories of useful and not useful. In fact their usefulness depends on individual circumstances and response to a supplement. Therefore, athletes can benefit from supplements:
* In situations with an unbalanced diet
* With specific alimentary conditions (e.g. vegan, lactose intolerance)
* In periods of weight reduction or "making weight"
* In periods with strenuous exercise and less time for recovery (e.g. training camps)
* While traveling in countries with limited food supply
* In some circumstances for some athletes (e.g. creatine, caffeine, buffering agents)

Finally:
* Sports dietitians should not ignore the importance of continuing their education in the field of sport nutrition and supplements.
* In addition, physicians, coaches, physiotherapists and parents need to be informed about the risks and benefits of DS as well

Chapter 14

Risks associated with dietary supplement use

Ronald Maughan

Supplement use

Dietary supplements are used by a substantial part of the general population, and the available evidence suggests that the rate of use is even higher among athletes (Huang et al. 2006). The pattern of use varies between sports and with the level of competition, but there can be few athletes who have not, at some stage in their career, taken dietary supplements. Most athletes are aware of the potential benefits of supplement use, and these benefits include the potential for health and performance enhancement (Maughan et al. 2007).

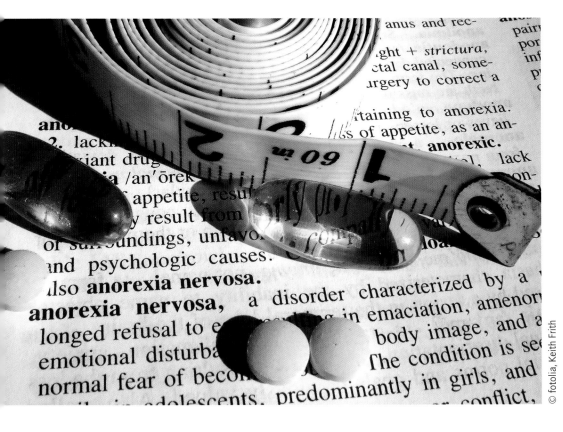

© fotolia, Keith Frith

Supplement regulation

Although there are undoubtedly benefits for some consumers of dietary supplements, there is also the potential for some negative outcomes. The Dietary Supplements Health and Education Act 1994 (DSHEA) passed by the US Congress has meant that nutritional supplements that do not claim to diagnose, prevent or cure disease are not subject to regulation by the Food and Drugs Administration (FDA). Supplements are regulated in the same way as food ingredients and are not subject to the stringent regulations that are applied to the pharmaceutical industry. From this it follows that there is no requirement to prove claimed benefits, no requirement to show safety with acute or chronic administration, no quality assurance and liberal labelling requirements. It is well recognized that there are problems with some of the dietary supplements on sale, but the options open to those responsible for food safety are limited by the legislation that applies. The FDA used its powers to recall a folic acid product because it was found to contain only 34% of the stated dose. They have also recently recalled products containing excessive doses of Vitamins A, D, B6 and selenium because of potentially toxic levels of these components. Some products have been shown to contain impurities (lead, broken glass, animal feces, etc.) because of the failure of the producers to observe good manufacturing practice. The risk of gastrointestinal upset because of poor hygiene during the production and storage of products is a concern to athletes. This may be nothing more than a minor inconvenience or it may cause the athlete to miss a crucial competition.

Quality control

Where the content of active ingredients in a supplement is variable, this is likely to be due to poor quality control during the manufacturing process. There is also evidence, however, that some products do not to contain an effective dose of expensive ingredients listed on the label, and in some cases, the active ingredient is entirely absent and the product contains only inexpensive materials. Even relatively inexpensive ingredients may be absent or present in only trivial amounts, as reported by Harris et al. (2004). This has been interpreted by some as a cost-saving exercise on the part of the manufacturers. A rather sophisticated chemical analysis is required to identify the contents of a supplement, so there is no way for athletes to know what is in any of these products.

Cost benefit analysis

Athletes who take supplements often have no clear understanding of the potential effects of the supplements they are using, but it seems clear that supplements should be used only after a careful cost-benefit analysis has been conducted. On one side of the balance are the rewards, the most obvious of which is an improved performance in sport, and on the other side lie the costs and the risks. Vitamin and mineral supplements are generally perceived as being harmless, and the one-a-day multivitamin tablet is seen as an insurance policy "just in case". Many herbal products are also used, even though there is little or no evidence to support their claimed benefits. The fact that most of these supplements enjoy only brief periods of popularity before disappearing from the marketplace suggests that any benefits perceived by athletes are not strong enough to warrant continued use or recommendation to friends and colleagues. Although these supplements are mostly benign, this is not always the case. Routine iron supplementation, for example, can do more harm than good, and the risk of iron toxicity is very real for many consumers.

Some supplements may actually cause harm to health, but these can be difficult to identify and are usually withdrawn only after a significant number of adverse events have occurred. In a recent case, a range of products containing hydroxycitric acid was withdrawn from sale, but only after they were linked with the death of one consumer and with a substantial number of other cases of liver toxicity, cardiovascular problems and seizures.

> Athletes who take supplements often have no clear understanding of the potential effects of the supplements they are using, but it seems clear that supplements should be used only after a careful cost-benefit analysis has been conducted.

Can a supplement cause a positive doping test?

The biggest concern for athletes, who are subject to testing for the use of drugs that are prohibited in sport, must be the possibility that a supplement may contain something that will cause a positive doping test (Maughan 2005). Only a very small number of individuals are tested for evidence of the use of doping agents, but these are invariably the most successful performers. For these athletes, a failed drugs test may mean the loss of medals won or records set, as well as temporary suspension from competition. It also leads to damage to the athlete's reputation and perhaps to permanent loss of employment and income. Where there has been deliberate cheating, such penalties seem entirely appropriate, but it is undoubtedly true that some failed doping tests can be attributed to the innocent ingestion of dietary supplements.

> Supplements may be contaminated and cause a positive doping test. There are even reports of several cases of serious adverse effects on health resulting from the use of dietary supplements containing undeclared anabolic steroids.

There are now numerous published studies to show that contamination of dietary supplements with prohibited substances is not uncommon (Maughan 2005). A wide range of stimulants, steroids and other agents that are included on the World Anti-Doping Agency's prohibited list has been identified in otherwise innocuous supplements. These instances are quite distinct from the legitimate sale of some of these substances, however, as their presence is not declared on the product label. In some cases these adulterated products are even labeled as being safe for use by athletes. In some, but not all, cases the extraneous additions have actions that are linked to the intended use of the product. Thus anabolic agents have been found in supplements sold as muscle growth promoters, stimulants in herbal tonics, and anorectic agents in herbal weight loss supplements. These observations suggest that this is either a deliberate act to add active ingredients to otherwise ineffective products or that the managers have allowed some mixing of separate products at the manufacturing facility. This might occur in the preparation of the raw ingredients or in the formulation of the finished product. In some cases, the amount of supplement present may be high, even higher than the normal therapeutic dose. Geyer et al. (2002) purchased a "body building" supplement in England and upon analysis found it to contain methandieneone (commonly known as Dianabol). This drug was present in high amounts, enough to have an anabolic effect, but also enough to produce serious side effects, including liver toxicity and carcinogenicity. Unlike many of the earlier cases involving steroids related to nandrolone and testosterone, this is not a trivial level of contamination and raises the possibility of deliberate adulteration of the product with the intention of producing a measurable effect on muscle strength and muscle mass. The prospect of adverse health effects at these high doses also raises real concerns. Recent reports have documented several cases of serious adverse effects on health resulting from the use of dietary supplements containing undeclared anabolic steroids (Krishnan 2009).

Can you guarantee a supplement is safe?

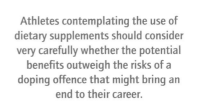

Athletes contemplating the use of dietary supplements should consider very carefully whether the potential benefits outweigh the risks of a doping offence that might bring an end to their career.

In spite of these problems, it is true that the majority of dietary supplements are safe and will not cause health problems or violations of the doping code. It is equally true, however, that a problem remains in that a significant minority of the products on sale to athletes carry such risks. Many attempts are being made to address these problems, but at present, there is no way in which a particular product can be guaranteed to be free of any risks. This is in part due to the extremely small amounts of some substances that may cause a positive doping outcome. Ingestion of 19-norandrostenedione, a prohibited substance and precursor of nandrolone, will result in its appearance in the urine, the diagnostic metabolite. If the urinary concentration of 19-norandrosterone exceeds 2 ng$\cdot$L^{-1}, a doping offence is deemed to have occurred. The addition of as little as 2.5μg of 19-norandrostenedione to a supplement, can result in a urinary concentration of 19-norandrosterone in excess of this threshold in some, but not all, individuals (Watson et al. 2009). This effect is transient, and it can be seen from Figure 1 that even when a larger dose (10μg) of steroid is administered, it is likely that only the first or second urine sample after ingestion will contain enough of the steroid metabolites to give a positive test. This means that an athlete who ingests this may or may not test positive, depending on when the sample is collected in relation to consumption of the supplement. The amount of steroid added is close to the limits of detection of the analytical methods currently applied to the analysis of dietary supplements, and there is no certainty that analysis of the finished product would have detected this.

The very small amounts of extraneous doping agents that have been reported to be present in many supplements – perhaps in as many as one in four of those selected for testing - will have no effect on physiological function, even though they may result in a positive doping test (Table 1; Geyer et al. 2004). It seems likely that their presence is due to accidental contamination at some stage of the manufacture, storage or distribution of the raw ingredients or of the finished product. This may be due to cross-contamination of production lines where prohibited substances are processed alongside dietary supplements or due to poor quality control in the production of raw ingredients.

Various efforts are being made to address the problems and to identify products that athletes may use with confidence. There can be no absolute guarantee that any product is entirely safe, but such schemes do help the athlete to manage the risk. Because of the strict liability principle that applies in doping cases, inadvertent ingestion of a prohibited substance through use of a contaminated dietary supplement does not absolve the athlete of guilt. Athletes contemplating the use of dietary supplements should consider very carefully whether the potential benefits outweigh the risks of a doping offence that might bring an end to their career.

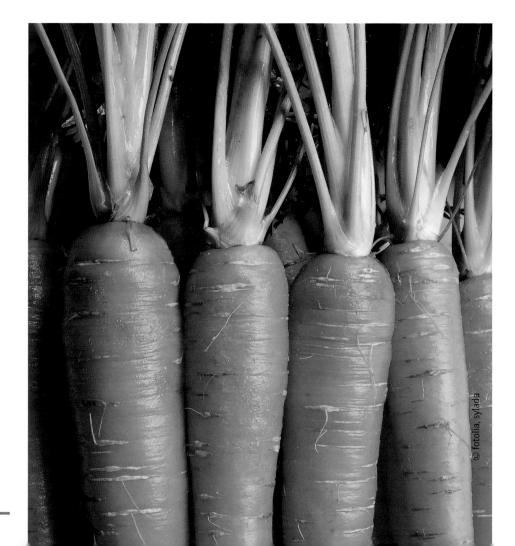

© fotolia, sylada

Table 1   Results of the analysis of dietary supplements for anabolic agents carried out for the International Olympic Committee by the Cologne Doping Laboratory (Geyer et al. 2004). For each country where supplements were purchased, the table shows the number of samples tested, the number that contained prohibited steroids and the fraction of the total this accounts for.

Country	No. tested	No. 'positive'	% 'positive'
Netherlands	31	8	25.8
Austria	22	5	22
UK	37	7	18.9
USA	240	45	18.8
Italy	35	5	14.3
Spain	29	4	13.8
Germany	129	15	11.6
Belgium	30	2	6.7
France	30	2	6.7
Norway	30	1	3.3
Switzerland	13	0	0
Sweden	6	0	0
Hungary	2	0	0
Total	634	94	14

Chapter 15

Nutrition and immune function

Michael Gleeson

Athletes at risk

There is some evidence that athletes who are training hard or who have recently competed in endurance race events are at increased risk of picking up minor illnesses and infections (Gleeson 2005). The most common illnesses in athletes are upper respiratory tract infections (URTI) the majority of which are caused by a virus rather than bacteria (and thus do not benefit from antibiotic therapy). In themselves, these episodes of URTI are generally trivial, but they can interrupt training or cause an athlete to miss (or under-perform in) important competitions.

Psychological stress, lack of sleep and malnutrition can depress immunity and lead to increased risk of infection.

Prolonged bouts of strenuous exercise, particularly if performed without carbohydrate intake, and periods of hard training with limited recovery and/or inadequate energy intake may compromise the body's immune system. In addition, high levels of stress hormones (e.g. cortisol, epinephrine/adrenaline) and anti-inflammatory cytokines (e.g. interleukins 6 and 10) brought on by chronic physical and/or psychological stress reduce the body's ability to fight opportunistic infections including colds and influenza. Acute bouts of strenuous aerobic exercise lasting 90 minutes or more have been shown to result in transient depression of several aspects of both innate and acquired immunity including decreased functional responses of monocytes, neutrophils, natural killer cells and T and B lymphocytes. It is suggested that such changes create an "open window" of decreased host protection, during which viruses and bacteria can gain a foothold, increasing the risk of developing an infection (Gleeson 2000; Nieman and Pedersen 2000). Other factors such as psychological stress, lack of sleep and malnutrition can also depress immunity and lead to increased risk of infection (Figure 1). There are also some situations in which an athlete's exposure to infectious agents may be increased.

Maintaining an effective immune system

Adequate nutrition and, in particular, appropriate intakes of energy, protein, vitamins and minerals are essential to maintain the body's natural defenses against disease causing micro-organisms (pathogens). Thus, athletes are best advised to consume a sound diet that meets their energy needs and contains a variety of foods. It is important to remember that any sustained deficiency of an essential vitamin or mineral will result in ill health (Calder et al. 2002) and it is extremely unlikely that an unhealthy athlete will perform to the best of his or her potential. Therefore, the key to maintaining an effective immune system is to avoid deficiencies of the nutrients that play an essential role in immune cell functions.

Inadequate protein-energy intake or deficiencies of certain micronutrients (e.g. iron, zinc and vitamins B6 and B12), decrease immune defenses against invading pathogens and make the individual more susceptible to infection (Calder et al. 2002; Gleeson et al. 2004). It is well accepted that an inadequate intake of protein impairs host immunity with particularly detrimental effects on the T-cell system, resulting in increased incidence of opportunistic infections. Essentially all forms of immunity have been shown to be affected by protein malnutrition in humans, depending on the severity of the protein deficiency relative to energy intake. While it is unlikely that athletes would ever reach a state of such extreme malnutrition unless dieting very severely or suffering from an eating disorder, some impairment of host defense mechanisms is observed even in moderate protein deficiency. In a study on judoists experiencing combined exercise and weight loss, significant falls in serum immunoglobulins and complement proteins were observed after only 4 weeks of dietary restriction that resulted in an average body mass loss of 2.8 kg (Umeda et al. 2004). In a similar study by the same researchers, falls in neutrophil function were also observed after a 20-

> Deficiencies of fat-soluble vitamins A and E and water-soluble vitamins folic acid, B6, B12 and C impair immune function and decrease the body's resistance to infection.

day period of combined exercise and dietary restriction (Yaegaki et al. 2007). Care should be taken to ensure adequate protein (and micronutrient) intakes during periods of intentional weight loss and it should be recognized that athletes undergoing weight reduction are more prone to infection.

Several vitamins are essential for normal immune function. Deficiencies of fat-soluble vitamins A and E and water-soluble vitamins folic acid, B6, B12 and C impair immune function and decrease the body's resistance to infection. Correcting existing deficiencies with specific vitamin supplements can be effective in restoring immune function to normal levels.

Several minerals are known to exert modulatory effects on immune function,

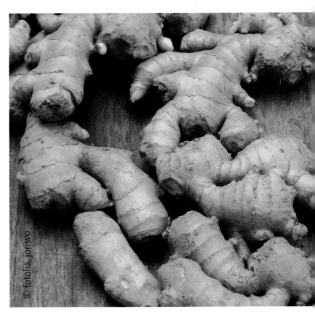

© fotolia, jorisvo

including zinc, iron, magnesium, manganese, selenium and copper, yet with the exception of zinc and iron, isolated deficiencies are rare. Field studies consistently associate iron deficiency with increased morbidity from infectious disease. Furthermore, exercise has a pronounced effect on both zinc and iron metabolism. Requirements for these minerals are certainly higher in athletes compared with sedentary people because of increased losses in sweat and urine. However, it is also recognized that excesses of iron and zinc can actually impair immune function. Hence, supplements should be taken only as required and regular monitoring of iron status (serum ferritin and blood hemoglobin) and zinc status (erythrocyte zinc) is probably a good idea.

Dietary surveys show that most athletes are well able to meet the recommended intakes for vitamins and minerals by eating everyday foods. Those at risk of sub-optimal intakes of these micronutrients include: (1) athletes who restrict their energy intake in an attempt to lose weight (fat), (2) athletes who follow eating patterns with restricted food variety and/or rely on foods with a poor micronutrient density. Especially when these practices are continued over long periods they can cause suboptimal intakes of micronutrients. In general, a broad-range multivitamin/mineral supplement is the best choice to support a restricted food intake, and this may also be suitable for the travelling athlete in situations where food choices and quality may be limited. It is also worth remembering that certain infections can also affect nutritional status by causing appetite suppression, malabsorption, increased losses of endogenous nutrients and increased nutrient requirements (Calder et al. 2002).

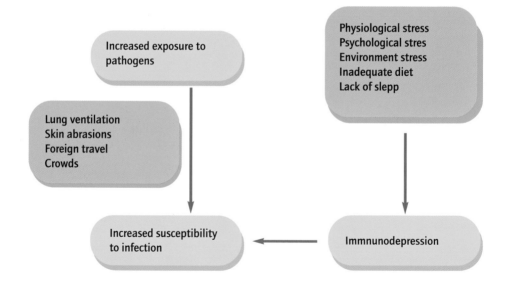

Figure 1: Causes of increased infection risk in athletes

Nutrition strategies to limit exercise-induced immune depression

Certain supplements may boost immune function and reduce infection risk in immune compromised individuals (Nieman and Pedersen 2000; Calder et al. 2002.). In fact, there are many nutritional supplements on the market with the claim that they boost immunity including: arginine, glutamine, bovine colostrum, whey protein, vitamin C, probiotics, zinc and herbals such as echinacea. However, such claims are often based on selective evidence of efficacy in animals, children, the elderly or clinical patients in severe catabolic states and in vitro experiments. Direct evidence for their efficacy for preventing exercise-induced immune depression or improving immune system status in athletes is usually lacking. A discussion of which immune-boosting supplements can be recommended for athletes can be found in the next chapter.

The best evidence supports the implementation of appropriate rest periods within the training micro-cycle and the use of a high carbohydrate diet and carbohydrate ingestion (about 30-60 grams per hour) during prolonged workouts, which lowers circulating epinephrine (adrenaline) and cortisol levels and delays the appearance of symptoms of overreaching during intensive training periods (Gleeson et al. 2004; Halson et al. 2004). Several placebo-controlled studies in runners and cyclists have shown that carbohydrate ingestion (usually in the form of a beverage) during prolonged exercise is effective in attenuating detrimental changes in some aspects of immune function (Gleeson 2006; Nieman 2008). However, evidence is currently lacking to demonstrate that this translates into a reduced incidence of URTI following competitive events.

The consumption of beverages during exercise not only helps prevent dehydration (which is associated with an increased stress hormone response) but also helps to maintain saliva flow rate during exercise. Saliva contains several proteins with antimicrobial properties including immunoglobulin A, lysozyme and a-amylase. Saliva secretion usually falls during exercise but regular fluid intake during exercise can prevent this (Bishop et al. 2000).

Relatively little is known about the potential contribution of dietary fatty acids to the regulation of exercise-induced modification of immune function. Two groups of polyunsaturated fatty acids (PUFA) are essential to the body: the omega-6 (n-6) series, derived from linoleic acid and the omega-3 (n-3) series, derived from linolenic acid. These PUFA cannot be synthesized in the body and therefore must be derived from the diet. There are reports that diets rich in either of these PUFA improve the conditions of patients

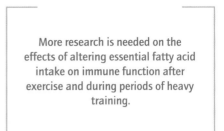

More research is needed on the effects of altering essential fatty acid intake on immune function after exercise and during periods of heavy training.

suffering from diseases characterized by an over-active immune system, such as rheumatoid arthritis; that is to say they have anti-inflammatory effects (Calder et al. 2002). Although no athletic study has been done yet, it is possible that an excessive intake of PUFA could further potentiate the exercise-induced depression of some immune cell functions. High intakes of arachidonic acid relative to intakes of PUFA of the n-3 group may also exert an undesirable influence on inflammation and immune function during and after exercise. More research is needed on the effects of altering essential fatty acid intake on immune function after exercise and during periods of heavy training.

Although it is not known whether hard training increases the need for dietary antioxidants – as the body naturally develops an effective defense with a balanced diet and endogenous antioxidant defenses actually improve with exercise training – some recent evidence suggests that regular intake of relatively high doses of antioxidant vitamins can also reduce the cortisol response to prolonged exercise (Halson et al. 2004; Gleeson, 2006). These studies have used combinations of vitamin C and E (Fischer et al. 2004), or vitamin C (Davison et al. 2006) alone, and provide a possible mechanism to explain earlier findings of a benefit of vitamin C supplementation in reducing the incidence of URTI symptoms in individuals who took part in ultramarathon races (Peters 2000). The body's tissue stores become saturated with regular vitamin C intakes of 200 mg·day[-1], so this amount, should in theory, be sufficient. Excessive supplementation with other antioxidants cannot be recommended because there is little evidence of benefit, while it is known that over-supplementation can actually diminish the body's natural antioxidant defense system and may even impair or diminish some adaptations to training. Ensuring that the diet contains plenty of fresh fruits and vegetables is probably the wisest option. However, nutrition is just one of a number of strategies that can help to reduce infection risk in athletes (see Table 1).

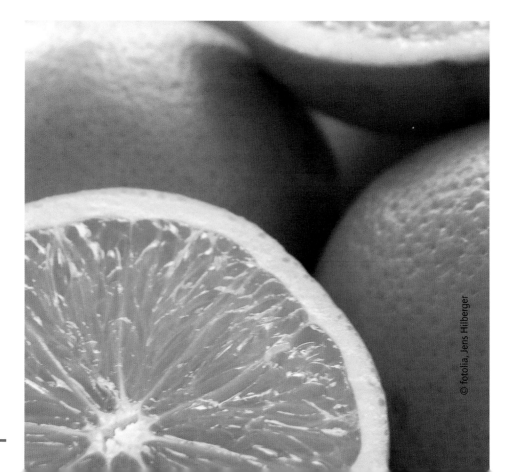

© fotolia, Jens Hilberger

Table 1: Strategies to counter illness risk in athletes

- Diet is important for immune function and many vitamins and minerals are associated with the ability to fight infection, particularly vitamin C, vitamin A and zinc. A good well-balanced diet should provide all the necessary vitamins and minerals, but if fresh fruit and vegetables are not readily available multivitamin supplements should be considered.
- Nutritional considerations should emphasize the need for adequate intakes of fluid, carbohydrate, protein and micronutrients. Ensuring the recovery of glycogen stores on a day-to-day basis and consuming carbohydrate during exercise (about 30-60 g of carbohydrate per hour during exercise seems to be effective) appear to be ways of minimizing the temporary immunodepression associated with an acute bout of prolonged exercise and reduces chances of developing overreaching symptoms.
- The evidence for the benefit of many so-called immune-boosting supplements (e.g. glutamine, echinacea, colostrum) is weak, though there is some evidence that probiotics and several antioxidant compounds (e.g. vitamin C, flavonoids such as quercetin) may be effective in reducing URTI risk.
- Avoid getting a dry mouth, both during competition and at rest; this can be done by drinking at regular intervals and maintaining hydration status.
- Never share drink bottles, cutlery or towels and use properly treated water for consumption.
- Other behavioral, lifestyle changes such as good hygiene practice (washing hands and brushing teeth regularly; using an antibacterial mouth rinse), may limit transmission of contagious illnesses by reducing exposure to common sources of infection.
- Avoid putting the hands to the eyes and nose (a major route of viral self-inoculation).
- Avoid overtraining and chronic fatigue.
- Keep other life/social/psychological stresses to a minimum (mental stress itself has been linked to depressed immunity and increased URTI risk).
- Get adequate sleep (minimum of 6 hours per day) on a regular schedule (sleep disruption has been linked to depressed immunity).
- Avoid rapid weight loss (this has been related to adverse immune changes). If some weight (fat) loss is desired, ensure adequate protein and micronutrient intake during periods of dietary energy restriction.
- Before important competitive events, avoid sick people and large crowds in enclosed spaces when possible.
- Medical support including regular checkups, appropriate immunization and prophylaxis may be particularly important for athletes who are at high risk of succumbing to recurrent infection.
- Vaccinate athletes and all support staff who are in regular contact with athletes.
- Be aware of particular vulnerability to infection after training or competition, especially in the winter months (this is when URTI are most prevalent in the general population).
- Training should be stopped if the athlete has a fever and/or systemic symptoms including aching joints and muscles. It is probably alright (and probably beneficial) to continue training (though at a reduced load) if the symptoms are all above the neck.
- Iron supplements should not be taken during periods of infection.
- Team members with infection should be isolated as much as possible from the rest of the team.

What all this means

In conclusion, strenuous bouts of prolonged exercise and heavy training stress the body both physically and mentally. For optimal health and performance it is particularly important to ensure adequate intakes of energy, carbohydrate, protein, calcium, copper, iron, magnesium, manganese, selenium, sodium, zinc and vitamins A, C, E, B6 and B12. These, and other nutrients, are best obtained from a varied and wholesome nutrient-rich diet based largely on vegetables, fruits, beans, legumes, grains, animal meats, oils and appropriate sources of carbohydrate (e.g. potatoes, bread, rice, pasta and cereals) for energy.

In general, a broad-range multivitamin/mineral supplement is the best choice to support a restricted food intake, or in situations where food choices and quality may be limited. If a particular micronutrient deficiency is identified such as iron deficiency, for example, a targeted short-term period of nutrient supplementation may be necessary. This should be undertaken in consultation with a qualified sports nutrition expert as over-supplementation with some micronutrients including vitamin E, iron and zinc can impair the body's immune defenses (Calder et al. 2002).

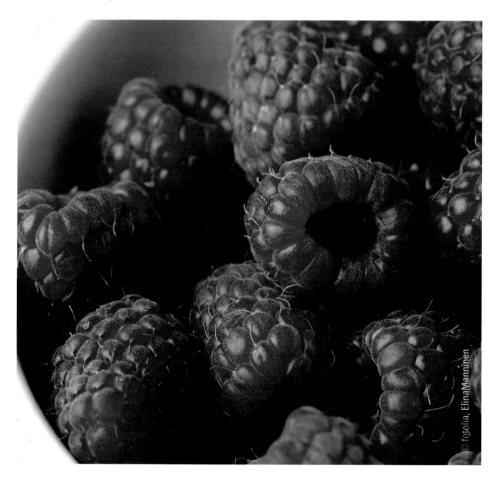

© fotolia, ElinaManninen

Chapter 16

Supplements to boost immune function

David Nieman

Introduction

Physical activity influences immune function and risk of certain types of infection such as upper respiratory tract infections (URTI). In contrast to moderate physical activity, prolonged and intensive exertion by endurance athletes causes numerous changes in immunity in multiple body compartments and an increased risk of URTI. Elite endurance athletes must train intensively to compete at the highest levels and are prime candidates for immunonutrition support to bolster immune system function in the face of physiological stress.

Influence of heavy exertion on immunity

Each acute bout of heavy exertion leads to physiological stress and transient, but clinically significant, changes in immunity and host pathogen defense. Since the early 1980s, it has been repeatedly shown that the immune system reflects the physiologic stress the endurance athlete's body is experiencing as circulating levels of stress hormones (e.g. cortisol, epinephrine/adrenaline),

> Epidemiological and exercise immunology studies support the viewpoint that heavy exercise workloads increase upper respiratory tract infection risk through altered immune function.

and pro- and anti-inflammatory cytokines (e.g. interleukins 6 and 10) rise to relatively high levels (Nieman 1997). Stress is also manifested by the suppression of certain immune parameters. Natural killer cell activity, various measures of T and B cell function, upper airway neutrophil function, salivary immunoglobulin A (IgA) concentration, granulocyte oxidative burst activity, skin delayed-type hypersensitivity response, and major histocompatibility complex (MHC) II and toll-like receptor expression in macrophages are suppressed for at least several hours during recovery from prolonged, intense endurance exercise. These immune changes occur in several compartments of the immune system and body (e.g., the skin, upper respiratory tract mucosal tissue, lung, blood, muscle, and peritoneal cavity).

Infection risk in athletes

Numerous studies have shown that several aspects of immune function are depressed for a period of time following a bout of prolonged strenuous exercise and this has been suggested to

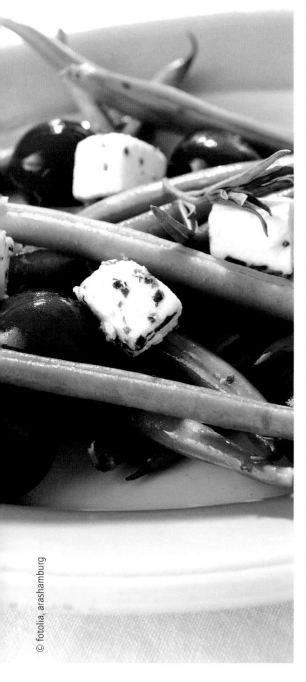

© fotolia, arashamburg

provide a potential "open window" for disease causing micro-organisms. During this "open window" of impaired immunity (which may last between 3 and 72 hours, depending on the immune measure), viruses and bacteria may gain a foothold, increasing the risk of subclinical and clinical infection. Several epidemiological studies have shown that athletes engaging in marathon and ultramarathon race events and/or very heavy training are at increased risk of URTI (Nieman 2000). Together, these epidemiological and exercise immunology studies support the viewpoint that heavy exercise workloads increase URTI risk through altered immune function.

Immunonutrition support for athletes

Various nutritional agents have been tested for their capacity to attenuate immune changes following intensive exercise and to lower the magnitude of physiologic stress and URTI risk. This strategy is similar to the immunonutrition support provided to patients recovering from trauma and surgery, and to the frail elderly. Supplements studied thus far in human athletes include: zinc, n-3 polyunsaturated fatty acids (n-3 PUFAs), plant sterols, antioxidants (e.g., vitamins C and E, beta-carotene, N-acetylcysteine, and butylated hydroxyanisole), glutamine, bovine colostrum, and carbohydrate (listed in Table 1). Immunonutrition support for athletes has been a major focus of research efforts of exercise immunologists during the past 15 years. Except for carbohydrate, results have been generally disappointing (see Table 1), and focus has shifted to examining the effects of probiotics and a new class of "advanced supplements" such as quercetin, isoquercetin, epigallocatechin 3-gallate (EGCG), β-glucan, and other plant polyphenols (Nieman 2008).

Table 1: Summary of rationale and findings for selected immunonutrition supplements.

Immunonutrition Supplement	Proposed Rationale	Recommendation Based On Current Evidence
n-3 PUFAs	Exerts anti-inflammatory effects post-exercise	Not recommended; no different from placebo
Vitamin E	Quenches exercise-induced reactive oxygen species (ROS) and augments immunity	Not recommended; may be pro-oxidative with heavy exertion.
Vitamin C	Quenches ROS and augments immunity Reduces cortisol response to exercise	Not recommended; relatively small effects on cortisol compared with carbohydrate; immune measures no different from placebo
Glutamine	Important immune cell energy substrate that is lowered with long exercise	Not recommended; body stores exceed exercise-lowering effects
Carbohydrate	Maintains blood glucose during exercise, lowers stress hormones, and thus counters immune dysfunction	Recommended, but 60 g·h of heavy exertion helps dampen immune inflammatory responses, but not all aspects of immune dysfunction.
β-glucan	Receptors found on immune cells, and animal data show supplementation improves innate immunity and reduces infection rates.	Not recommended; human study with athletes showed no benefits.
Echinacea	Herbal extract that is a popular supplement among athletes. Claimed to boost immunity via stimulatory effects on macrophages and there is some in vitro evidence for this.	Not recommended; large scale human study showed no benefits.
Probiotics	Probiotics are live microorganisms which when administered orally for several weeks, can increase the numbers of beneficial bacteria in the gut. This has been associated with a range of potential benefits to gut health, as well as modulation of immune function.	Recommended; human studies show improvements in some aspects of acquired immunity and reduced incidence of respiratory illness and gastrointestinal problems.
Quercetin	In vitro studies show strong anti-inflammatory, anti-oxidative, and anti-pathogenic effects. Animal data indicate increase in mitochondrial biogenesis and endurance performance.	Recommended; human studies show strong reduction in illness rates during heavy training and mild stimulation of mitochondrial biogenesis and endurance performance in untrained subjects.
Quercetin with EGCG	Flavonoid mixture promotes anti-inflammatory and anti-oxidative effects, and immune function improvement, superior to just quercetin alone.	Recommended; human study showed strong anti-inflammatory effect, with modest anti-oxidative effect and improvement in innate immunity.

Carbohydrate: A partial countermeasure

Carbohydrate beverage ingestion during prolonged exercise (about one liter/hour of a 6% carbohydrate beverage – typical of many sports drinks) attenuates increases in blood neutrophil and monocyte counts, stress hormones, and anti-inflammatory cytokines such as IL-6, IL-10, and IL-1ra and it prevents falls in T cell cytokine (e.g. interferon-gamma) production. There is little effect on decrements in salivary IgA output and natural killer cell function (Nieman and Bishop 2006). Thus, carbohydrate ingestion during heavy exercise has emerged as an effective, though partial, countermeasure to immune dysfunction, with favorable effects on measures related to stress hormones and inflammation, but with limited effects on the downturns in innate or adaptive immunity.

Probiotics: evidence of benefit to athletes

In recent years a few studies have examined the efficacy of oral probiotics in athletes and some of these have shown some promise (Gleeson 2008). Often called the friendly bacteria, probiotics are live microorganisms which when administered in adequate amounts, modify the intestinal microbiota such that the numbers of beneficial bacteria increase and generally numbers of species considered harmful are decreased. This has been associated with a range of potential benefits to gut health, as well as modulation of immune function by their interaction with the gut-associated lymphoid tissue, leading to positive effects on the systemic immune system. Some placebo-controlled studies in athletes have indicated that daily probiotic ingestion results in fewer days of respiratory illness and lower severity of URTI symptoms (Gleeson and Thomas 2008). In one study this was associated with a significant increase in whole blood culture interferon-gamma production, which may be one mechanism underpinning the positive clinical outcomes (Cox et al. 2008).

Advanced nutritional supplements

In vitro/cell culture and animal research indicate that advanced supplements such as ,-glucan, curcumin, quercetin, isoquercetin, EGCG, and other plant polyphenols warrant human investigations to determine if they are effective countermeasures to exercise-induced immune dysfunction and risk of URTI. Our evolving hypothesis is that the immune system is so diverse that a cocktail of these advanced supplements within a carbohydrate beverage will probably perform better than any single one alone. Some recent research has affirmed this approach (Nieman et al. 2009). Most benefit is likely to accrue from supplements that primarily target the nonspecific, innate arm of the immune system to enhance immunosurveillance against a wide variety of pathogens.

> Some placebo-controlled studies in athletes have indicated that daily probiotic ingestion results in fewer days of respiratory illness and lower severity of URTI symptoms.

β-Glucan: Impressive data in mice but not humans

β-Glucans are polysaccharides found in the bran of oat and barley cereal grains, the cell wall of baker's yeast, certain types of fungi, and many kinds of mushrooms. Evidence from studies conducted with rodents, fish, poultry, and swine indicates that oral ,-glucan ingestion stimulates innate immune defenses and antitumor responses, and increases resistance to a wide variety of infections. Rodent studies indicate that oat ,-glucan supplements offset the increased risk of infection associated with exercise stress through augmentation of macrophage and neutrophil function.

In a recent human athlete trial of this supplement (Nieman et al. 2008) the results were not so impressive. A double-blinded, placebo-controlled study was conducted on cyclists who received 5.6 g·day^{-1} of oat β-glucan or placebo beverage supplements for two weeks prior to, during, and one day after a 3-day period in which subjects cycled for 3 h·day^{-1} at 57% Wattsmax. The oat β-glucan supplement did not alter chronic resting or exercise-induced changes in immune function or URTI incidence in the cyclists during the 2-week period following intensified exercise (Nieman et al. 2008). This study is a useful reminder that nutritional supplements that work in mice often do not confer similar benefits in human subjects.

Quercetin

The physiologic effects of dietary flavonols such as quercetin are of great current interest due to their antioxidative, anti-inflammatory, anti-pathogenic, cardioprotective, and anticarcinogenic activities. The richest food sources of quercetin are onions, apples, blueberries, curly kale, hot peppers, tea, and broccoli. Total flavonol intake (with quercetin representing about 75%) varies from 13 to 64 mg·day^{-1} depending on the study sample and the population studied. Human subjects can absorb significant amounts of quercetin from food or supplements, and elimination is quite slow, with a reported half-life ranging from 11-28 hours. Animal studies indicate that 7-days quercetin feeding augments muscle and brain mitochondrial biogenesis, endurance performance, and survival from influenza virus inoculation.

A double-blind, placebo-controlled study with 40 cyclists showed that 1,000 mg·day^{-1} quercetin for three weeks significantly increased plasma quercetin levels and reduced URTI incidence during the 2-week period following 3-days of exhaustive exercise (Nieman et al. 2007). (Figure 1). Immune dysfunction, inflammation, and oxidative stress, however, were not altered suggesting that quercetin exerted direct anti-viral effects, at least within the context of the study design. Mitochondrial biogenesis was not increased following the 3-week period of quercetin supplementation in the trained cyclists. However, a follow-up study with untrained subjects showed a significant increase in endurance performance and an increase in mtDNA, but not nearly to the extent seen in mice following quercetin feeding.

There is increasing support for coingestion of quercetin with other flavonoids and food components to improve and extend quercetin's bioavailability and bioactive effects. These

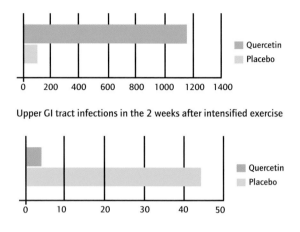

Plasma quercetin after 3 weeks of supplementation

Upper GI tract infections in the 2 weeks after intensified exercise

Figure 1 Plasma quercetin levels (P<0.001) and upper respiratory tract infection (URTI) infection rates (P=0.004) in cyclists during a 2-week period following a 3-day period of overtraining and ingestion of quercetin (1,000 mg·day^{-1}) or placebo (9).

include: the flavonoid EGCG from tea, isoquercetin which is the glycosylated form of quercetin in onions and other foods, n-3-polyunsaturated fatty acids (n-3-PUFAs) such as eicosapentaenoic acid (EPA) and docosahexaenoic acid (DHA), and the nutrients vitamin C and folate. In a study with 39 trained cyclists, a quercetin supplement combined with EGCG, isoquercetin, and n-3-PUFAs was more effective than quercetin alone in partially countering exercise-induced inflammation and oxidative stress (Nieman et al. 2007). These data add to a growing literature support for the concept that quercetin's anti-inflammatory and anti-oxidative effects are amplified when combined, in supplement form, with other flavonoids, food components, and micronutrients.

> There is increasing support for coingestion of quercetin with other flavonoids and food components to improve and extend quercetin's bioavailability and bioactive effects.

Final remarks

Endurance athletes must train hard for competition and are interested in strategies to keep their immune systems robust and to avoid illness despite the physiologic stress they experience. The ultimate goal is to provide athletes with a sports drink containing carbohydrate and a cocktail of advanced supplements that will lower infection risk, exert significant and measurable influences on their innate immune systems, and attenuate exercise-induced oxidative stress and inflammation. The athlete can combine this strategy with consumption of probiotic supplements that may convey some benefit to acquired immunity, reduce infection incidence and URTI symptom severity as well as reducing gastrointestinal problems.

Chapter 17

Sports nutrition for women

Brent Ruby

Introduction

Are men different from women? A quick search command from the pivotal world of Google generates 319 million results. How the sexes may differ in "fuel metabolism" captures only about $1/2$ of a percent of Google's attention. The primary discussions on how the sexes are similar and inherently different mingle in cyberspace and hover between psychology, workplace politics, learning patterns, social concerns. The list continues to grow.

In her 2005 book entitled, "Why Men Never Remember and Women Never Forget," Marianne Legato recognizes some of the key ingredients that underline the differences between the sexes.

> "In other words, our genes set us up for the sex we'll be, and our hormones salt the stew. The complex interaction between these two factors—especially during specific windows when their levels drop or surge as they do during puberty and menopause—make the two sexes different and each of us different from one another as well."

The primary focus of this discussion will include characteristics of fuel metabolism that can be altered by the "salt of the stew" and how these differences may be more prominent or suppressed at different stages of the life cycle. Additional attention will be directed to some of the methodology surrounding the measurement of muscle fuel use, the biological significance of sex-specific metabolic patterns, food fuels during muscle work and recovery and how this transitions to the world outside of the laboratory. Since most research is based on findings in men the main question is, Should the advice for women be different than the advice we give to men?

Anatomy, physiology, and research design

Basic anatomy reveals unique sex characteristics rooted in biological significance and function. However, the impact of sex on the underlying physiology offers more subtle differences at the cellular level during the selection, mobilization, and subsequent oxidation of muscle fuels during exercise. Although the data presented in Figure 1 represents a relatively small sample size (n=5 males, n=8 females), it shows the relative contribution of the dominant endogenous substrates available to the skeletal muscles of both sexes during moderate intensity exercise (65% if VO_2peak). Both sexes rely heavily on fuels within the muscle as well as plasma free fatty acids (FFA).

These data suggest that the mechanisms by which unique sex characteristics exert control over the use of muscle substrates are less influential compared to the dominant effects of training status and dietary state. The combination and relative contribution of these fuels to the working muscle during varying intensities and durations of exercise offers a near limitless series of metabolic choices. This combination is further influenced and altered by the introduction of exogenous fuel sources, which may provide a large portion of muscle substrate during extended work and exercise settings.

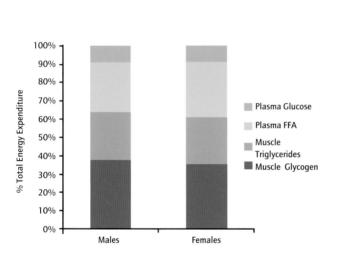

Figure 1. Estimated relative contribution of endogenous muscle substrates oxidized at 65% of VO$_2$peak. Data adapted from Romijn et al. (1993, 2000). Relative contribution data generated from indirect calorimetry and stable isotope infusion ([6,6 ^{2}H$_2$] glucose and [^{2}H$_2$] palmitate.

The majority of recent sex comparison studies evaluate similarly trained or tightly matched subjects (based on a series of criteria associated with current fitness levels and training/ competition histories) in a fasted state. In a recent review article, Tarnopolsky compares the data from 25 studies using meta-analyses and demonstrates a lower RER (indicating higher relative contribution of fat to total energy expenditure) for females compared to males (0.87 and 0.90 for females and males, respectively). These data pool a variety of exercise protocols (with an exercise duration >60 min.) and approaches to subject selection. From these data, it appears that females demonstrate a higher fat oxidation compared to males during moderate intensity exercise. However, the underlying significance from a biological and/or exercise performance/work perspective remains somewhat unclear.

Additional insight can be gained from the literature investigating metabolic differences in children and adolescents. Timmons et al. (2007) have demonstrated that younger girls (aged 12 y) show a higher rates of fat oxidation compared to older girls (aged 14 y), an apparent influence of the stages of puberty. How this may help explain sex differences in young adults (aged 18 y) versus more mature endurance athletes (aged 25-35 y) remains unclear.

It appears that females demonstrate a higher fat oxidation compared to males during moderate intensity exercise.

However, in response to the rigors of regular exercise training, the reproductive hormones that strongly influence female sex characteristics ebb and flow as a function of energy intake and balance. From a biological standpoint, preservation of select endogenous substrates and shifting substrate use profiles provide advantages to fetal development should pregnancy occur.

To eat or not to eat during exercise?

It has been suggested that because females have demonstrated a lower dependence on muscle glycogen during 90 minutes of moderate intensity exercise (Tarnopolsky 1990), that they may excel in endurance and ultra-endurance events. However, to perform at a high level during these events, careful approaches to exogenous intake behavior are imperative. Therefore, it is unclear whether a slightly higher fat oxidation would provide clear benefits during extended work settings where exogenous intake becomes mandatory to maintain work output.

Wallis et al. (2006) evaluated the metabolic responses in similarly trained men and women during 2 hours of continuous cycling exercise (67% VO_2peak) with and without exogenous carbohydrate (CHO). During the trials, subjects consumed equal volumes of CHO or water at regular intervals. Carbohydrate was consumed at a rate of 90 g·h^{-1} throughout the exercise. Exogenous CHO increased total CHO oxidation for both males and females and reached similar peak rates of oxidation (approximately 0.6 g·min^{-1}). Overall, these data indicate that although exogenous carbohydrate intake suppresses the use of endogenous fuels (liver glycogen and whole body fat); the responses between the sexes are similar (Figure 2). Moreover, these data are similar to those reported by M'Kaouar et al. (2004) and Riddell et al. (2003) and suggest that both males and females may benefit equally from similar exogenous feeding schedules during extended exercise/work settings.

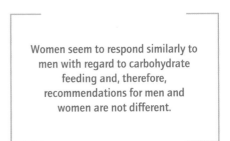
Women seem to respond similarly to men with regard to carbohydrate feeding and, therefore, recommendations for men and women are not different.

Although the idea of suggesting similar intake patterns for males and females simplifies the calculations, the need for individual trial and error should not be understated. For a 72 kg male, an intake of 60g·h^{-1} would amount to 0.8 g·kg^{-1}·h^{-1} compared to a 55 kg female (1.1 g·kg^{-1}·h^{-1}), a difference that may result in significant stomach discomfort in the smaller female. However, the trainability of the GI system to tolerate and accept exogenous CHO should also not be discounted. This requires further attention as it relates to maximizing the rate of exogenous CHO oxidation. This is especially true during towards the end of extended bouts of muscle work during which the exogenous intake may provide a nearly 100%very large percentage of the CHO fuel for total CHO oxidation.

During a 10-hour intermittent exercise trial in our laboratory (Harger-Domitrovich et al. 2007), males (n=7) and females (n=6) were provided with exogenous CHO or placebo. Net muscle glycogen use was 52% higher during the placebo trial. However, there were no differences

■ Exogenous CHO   ■ Liver CHO   ■ Muscle CHO   ■ FAT

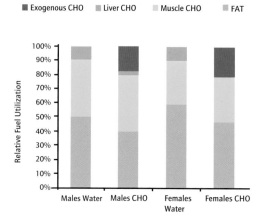

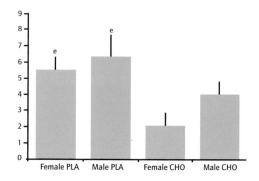

Figure 2. The relative contribution of endogenous and exogenous substrate oxidation during exercise. Adapted from Wallis et al. (2006).

Figure 3. Muscle glycogen breakdown for the two exercise trials. e=p<0.05 vs. CHO trial for males and females. Main effect for trial. Adapted from Harger-Domitrovich (2007).

between the sexes (Figure 3). Under these conditions (extended exercise), exogenous CHO accounts for a large percentage of the total CHO oxidation and reduces the demand placed on endogenous CHO sources (liver and muscle glycogen) regardless of sex.

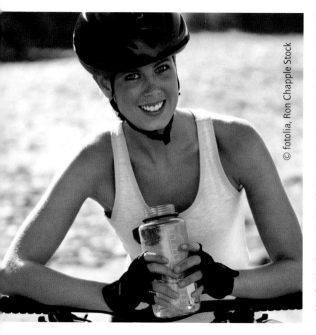

© fotolia, Ron Chapple Stock

Glycogen loading and recovery

Although past data suggests that males and female derive similar benefits from exogenous CHO consumed at similar rates, the ability to better prepare for endurance competitions through CHO loading may be somewhat limited to males. Tarnopolsky et al. (1995) showed that females were not able to increase muscle glycogen via traditional approaches to CHO loading. In contrast, if CHO intake can be increased to >8.0 $g \cdot kg^{-1} \cdot day^{-1}$, glycogen can be pre-loaded into the female muscle. However, this approach may be less practical for females due to the high % of CHO required to achieve super compensation (usually >70% of total energy intake). These data place further importance on maximizing the system's ability to tolerate higher rates of exogenous CHO sources during the period of exercise/work.

In response to glycogen depleting exercise, Tarnopolsky et al. (1997) showed that a CHO or a CHO-protein source enhanced glycogen recovery similarly in males and females. This early approach to recovery may be recommended for both sexes if additional training periods/competitions are scheduled for later that day or the next.

Sex comparisons outside of the typical laboratory

Collectively, the literature suggests that there are testing situations in the laboratory where males and females differ in the selection and oxidation of muscle substrates. These observations are essential for understanding the basic biological significance the sex hormones have with regard to development and reproduction. However, when transitioned outside of the laboratory, the subtle sex differences in the fasted state and the unique control exerted by the sex specific hormones become less influential than the required dietary and environmental adjustments necessary to sustain muscle work in the field. In these settings, sex is put aside and the hostilities of the environment dictate the required response.

> When compared under extended field exercise conditions, subtle differences in metabolism are diminished and there are limited differences between males and females.

During the 2005/2006 Ironman World Championships in Kona, Hawaii and during the 2007 Western States 100 ultramarathon, our laboratory quantified total energy expenditure (TEE) of competitors (doubly labeled water). In Kona, TEE was 9,253 and 9,920 kcals for the two male subjects and 8,238 kcals for the female. Relative to total body weight TEE for the female (135 kcals·kg^{-1}) was slightly higher compared to the males (119 and 122 kcals·kg^{-1}, respectively). For a 10-hour race, considering an average intake of 60 g·h^{-1}, exogenous CHO and total energy intake may account for approximately 25-30% of the TEE.

Similarly, during the Western States 100, males and females were evaluated for measures of TEE and water turnover (rH2O). Although males were significantly heavier (78.4±8.0 kg) compared to females (61.5±7.7 kg), there were no differences in finish times (26.4±2.9 and 27.1±3.7 hours) or total energy expenditure (221±23 and 228±23 kcals·kg^{-1}·race^{-1} for males and females, respectively). Calculated rates of water turnover were also similar for both sexes (254±37 and 259±49 ml·kg^{-1}·race^{-1} for males and females, respectively).

Conclusions

Laboratory data demonstrates a tendency for females to oxidize more whole body fat in comparison to similarly trained males. The majority of these differences appear to be the result

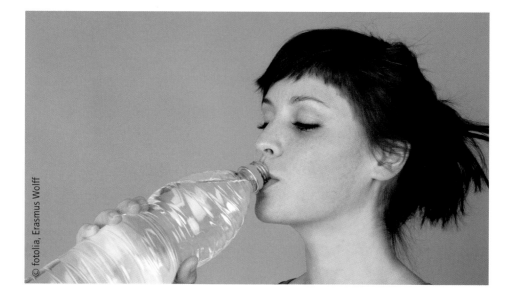

© fotolia, Erasmus Wolff

of 17-β estradiol and the influence it exerts on the mRNA of human skeletal muscle. These subtle alterations can influence fat, CHO and protein metabolism to ensure a sex-specific metabolism that asserts biological significance to ensure an ideal in vivo environment for reproductive health. The extent to which these subtle variations may influence extended muscle work or endurance competition is uncertain. However, it appears that the effects of exogenous CHO on substrate oxidation are similar for both males and females. Moreover, when compared under extended field exercise conditions, subtle differences in metabolism are diminished and there are limited differences between males and females. Therefore, there is no reason to believe that the nutrition advice given to females should be different than the advice given to males.

Table 1

Nutritional intervention	Rate	Physiological Response	Benefit
None	- - -	females > fat oxidation	?
Exogenous CHO during	1-1.5* g·min⁻¹	maximize CHO availability preserve endogenous CHO (liver, muscle?)	>power output >output longer
CHO during recovery	1 g·kg⁻¹CHO @0, 60min post	> glycogen resynthesis	>recovery for next session/ competition

1.5 g.min⁻¹ only recommended when a mixture of carbohydrates is ingested i.e. glucose+fructose

Chapter 18

Nutrition, the brain and prolonged exercise

Romain Meeusen and Phil Watson

The brain (central nervous system; CNS) is the 'cockpit' where decisions are made and from where signals to the muscles originate to produce the movements required to perform exercise. This cockpit is often referred the "centre", the muscles are referred to as the "periphery". The brain and periphery are constantly communicating; the periphery informs the brain about its metabolic needs and the brain provides for these needs through its control of (somatomotor, autonomic, and neurohumoral) pathways involved in energy intake, expenditure and storage.

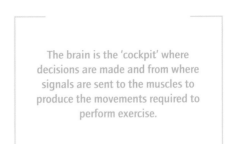

The brain is the 'cockpit' where decisions are made and from where signals are sent to the muscles to produce the movements required to perform exercise.

Events arising entirely from within the brain can influence an individual's sensation of fatigue and thus potentially affect performance. This opens an opportunity to manipulate the central nervous system through changes in diet or supplementation with specific nutrients, including amino acids (branched-chain amino acids, tyrosine), carbohydrates and caffeine. Some nutritional supplements that may influence performance during prolonged exercise are outlined in Table 1.

The original central fatigue hypothesis

The constant interaction between the brain and the periphery is present at rest but also during prolonged exercise. It has been hypothesized that a disturbance in the communication could be the cause of fatigue. This disturbance could be caused by a change in the signal transduction (by neurotransmitters) as a result of changes in the provision of neurotransmitter precursors. The original central fatigue hypothesis suggested that changes in the mobilization of substrates (CHO, fat) that occurs during exercise produces a direct effect on the production of the neurotransmitter serotonin (also called 5-HT) within the brain. Serotonin has been linked to fatigue because of its well-known effects on sleep, lethargy and loss of motivation. An exercise-induced increase in extracellular serotonin concentrations in several brain regions was suggested to contribute to the development of fatigue during prolonged exercise. Several nutritional and pharmacological studies have attempted to manipulate central serotonergic activity during exercise, but this work has yet to provide robust evidence for a significant role of serotonin in the fatigue process.

Nutrition and central fatigue

It was hypothesized that by reducing the production of serotonin in the brain, feelings of fatigue could be attenuated and performance enhanced. Supplementation of branched chain amino acids (BCAA) has been proposed as a possible strategy to limit the development of central fatigue. BCAA compete with the precursor of serotonin (tryptophan) for transport across the blood brain barrier. If more BCAAs are available in the circulation, then more will be transported across the blood brain barrier at the cost of tryptophan. This would imply that with increased BCAA availability, less tryptophan will be available in the brain, less serotonin would be formed, and, consequently, fatigue would be reduced. Although this is a very attractive theory, there is limited or only circumstantial evidence to suggest that exercise performance can be

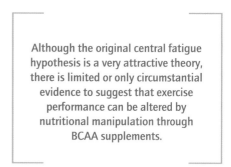

Although the original central fatigue hypothesis is a very attractive theory, there is limited or only circumstantial evidence to suggest that exercise performance can be altered by nutritional manipulation through BCAA supplements.

altered by nutritional manipulation through BCAA supplements. While there is some evidence of BCAA ingestion influencing ratings of perceived exertion and mental performance, the results of several well-controlled laboratory studies have failed to demonstrate a positive effect on exercise capacity or performance (Meeusen and Watson 2007).

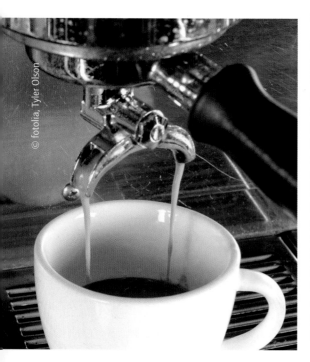

© fotolia, Tyler Olson

Caffeine

Caffeine has long been recognized as an ergogenic aid. It is one of the substances that lies in the grey area between a nutrition supplement and drugs. For a while, caffeine use was restricted by athletes, and it was only removed from the list of banned substances in January 2004 and put on the monitoring list. It has been shown to improve performance in events that last as short as 2-3 min up to very prolonged events. Although originally a metabolic explanation was preferred, it is now evident that the effect of caffeine is almost entirely mediated through its stimulant effect on the CNS. Caffeine acts as adenosine antagonist, essentially blocking the adenosine activity within the brain. As adenosine inhibits excitatory neural activity, caffeine reduces the action of adenosine and consequently increases neural activity.

Caffeine seems to be especially potent in events that require exercise at 70-80%VO$_2$max, while also producing marked effects on alertness, decision making and other cognitive functions. Caffeine has been shown to be effective in relatively low doses (2-3 mg·kg^{-1}) and its effect seems to level off at 5 mg·kg^{-1}. Therefore, it is not recommended to take very high doses. Given the widespread use of caffeine by many, the level of habitual intake may be an important factor to consider when using caffeine supplementation to enhance performance. In some individuals, who are unaccustomed to caffeine, caffeine can produce several side effects, such as tachycardia and palpitations, nervousness, dizziness and gastro-intestinal symptoms that may be detrimental to performance. The positive (and possible negative) effects of caffeine seem very individually determined so prior experience with doses and timing is essential before using supplementation in competitive environments.

> Caffeine seems to be especially potent in events that require exercise at 70-80%VO$_2$max, while also producing marked effects on alertness, decision making and other cognitive functions.

Carbohydrate

Another nutritional strategy that may influence the development of central fatigue is carbohydrate (CHO) feeding. The ingestion of CHO suppresses lipolysis, lowering the circulating concentration of plasma fatty acids and consequently limiting the exercise-induced rise in free-tryptophan. Recent work has demonstrated that CHO ingestion during exercise attenuated the cerebral uptake of tryptophan and prevented the development of hypoglycemia as well, though this does not rule out the peripheral role of CHO ingestion. The beneficial effect of CHO supplementation during prolonged exercise could also relate to increased (or maintained) substrate delivery for the brain. A number of studies indicate that hypoglycemia affects brain function and cognitive performance. Glucose is the only fuel for the brain so if the availability is reduced it is not unexpected that its function is impaired.

> Besides a metabolic effect of carbohydrate, especially during very prolonged exercise, carbohydrate may also have effects on the brain that enhance exercise performance lasting approximately 1 hour.

Carbohydrate feeding has been shown to improve exercise performance lasting approximately 60 min even though the estimated amount of glucose delivered to the muscle during this period was estimated to be very small (Jeukendrup et al. 1997). The same research group infused glucose during a time trial to study the performance effects with increased carbohydrate availability. Failure to observe a benefit of glucose infusion on time trial performance (Carter et al. 2004a), prompted this group to suggest an alternative mechanism for the ergogenic effect of CHO centered around the activation of CHO receptors found in the mouth. Carter et al. (2004b) reported a 3% (PLA 61.37 min; CHO 59.57 min) increase in performance following the rinsing of a maltodextrin solution around the mouth before and during exercise. No solution was actually ingested during the protocol, suggesting that this performance benefit may have been mediated through direct communication between receptors present in the mouth and the brain. This concept has been supported by work investigating brain activity following the ingestion of a bolus of glucose (Liu et al. 2000) and research demonstrating activation of several brain regions after rinsing CHO solutions within the mouth (Chambers et al. 2009). These studies highlight a marked increase in brain activation, occurring immediately after CHO enters the mouth, with a second spike in activity observed 10 minutes following ingestion, presumably occurring as the substrate enters the circulation. These findings are very novel and suggest an interesting mechanism of action. Further investigation of CHO receptors in the mouth is certainly warranted.

Other central mechanisms

Events that take place in the brain are dependent on neurotransmitters. It is important to note that brain function is not determined by a single neurotransmitter system. The interaction between brain serotonin and dopamine during prolonged exercise has also been explored for its possible regulative role in the development of fatigue. This revised central fatigue hypothesis suggests that an increase in central ratio of serotonin to dopamine is associated with feelings of tiredness and lethargy, accelerating the onset of fatigue, whereas a low ratio favors improved performance through the maintenance of motivation and arousal. Convincing evidence for a role of dopamine in the development of fatigue comes from work investigating the physiological responses to drugs which manipulate central catecholamine release (Roelands et al. 2008; Watson et al. 2005).

Despite a good rationale for the use of tyrosine, evidence of an ergogenic benefit of tyrosine supplementation during prolonged exercise is limited.

Increased catecholaminergic neurotransmission will favor feelings of arousal, motivation and reward, consequently enhancing exercise performance. In a similar manner to serotonin, brain dopamine and noradrenaline synthesis is reliant on the delivery of the non-essential amino acid tyrosine, but the rate of production appears to be also limited by the activity of the catecholaminergic neurons. Oral doses of tyrosine increase circulating concentrations of epinephrine, norepinephrine, and dopamine, both in the CNS and periphery. These are heavily involved in the regulation of body function during physical stress and exercise. Tyrosine appears to prevent declines in various aspects of cognitive performance and mood associated with stress encountered in some military settings (Lieberman 2003). There is some evidence that vigilance, choice reaction time, pattern recognition, coding and complex behaviors (such as map-compass reading) are improved by tyrosine administration when volunteers are exposed to the combination of cold and high altitude. The implications for the sports performer remain unclear. Despite a good rationale for its use, evidence of an ergogenic benefit of tyrosine supplementation during prolonged exercise is limited (Meeusen and Watson 2007). It is also worth noting that regular supplementation of large amounts of tyrosine (5 g to 10 g) may have adverse health effects due to chronic changes in sympathetic nervous system activity.

Table 1: Effects of supplements that act on the central nervous system

Supplement	Dose(s) studied	Proposed effect on the brain	Does it influence performance?
Branched-chain amino acids (BCAA)	5-20g	Reduces brain serotonin production	• Evidence is generally weak. • A few studies suggest an effect, but many more find no benefit. • May reduce perception of effort and enhance mental performance during exercise
Caffeine	2-10 mg·kg^{-1} BM	Reduces effect of adenosine in the brain	• Performance in events lasting more than a couple of minutes can be enhanced by caffeine. • Alters mood, increases alertness and reaction times • Large individual variation in sensitivity to caffeine
Carbohydrate (CHO)	30-90g·h^{-1}	Increased energy for the brain. Influences neurotransmission and cerebral metabolism	• Evidence suggests a benefit to performance in most cases. • Possible that part of this ergogenic effect is due to influence on the CNS
Tyrosine	5-10g	Increases production of brain dopamine and noradrenaline	• Few studies investigating effect of tyrosine on performance, but show no effect on physical performance

Some evidence of a benefit to mood, memory and cognitive function

Conclusions

Fatigue is a complex and multifaceted phenomenon. Much of the attraction of the original central fatigue hypothesis was the potential for nutritional manipulation of neurotransmitter precursors to delay the onset of central fatigue and potentially enhance performance. However several studies have found no effect of amino acid supplementation (BCAA, tyrosine) on a number of measures of exercise performance. There is good evidence that carbohydrate and caffeine can enhance performance in a variety of exercise situations and recent findings suggest that the CNS plays a key role in these responses.

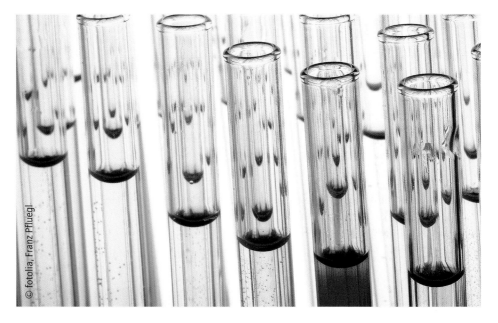

© fotolia, Franz Pfluegl

Some points for consideration when using supplements to influence the development of central fatigue

- This is a relatively new area of research in exercise physiology, and there are still many gaps in our knowledge of the effects of these supplements.
- At the moment, consistent benefits to performance during prolonged exercise are only reported with caffeine or carbohydrate.
- This is not to say that amino acid may not be useful. There is some emerging evidence that various aspects of mental fatigue and cognitive function can be positively influenced. In sports requiring the controlled execution of skills and/or rapid decision making, amino acid supplements may yet prove beneficial.
- Everyone is different and individuals may experience varying responses to some of these supplements. This is particularly apparent when considering caffeine supplementation: some experience marked effects with small doses, while others display little noticeable effects, even with relatively large amounts. For this reason it is advised that these supplements are used first in training, ahead of competition.
- Some supplement manufactures have jumped on results of early studies and introduced products with ingredients that claim to delay 'mental fatigue' (e.g. BCAAs). Often the inclusion of these ingredients is done with little sound evidence and the amount of the ingredient included is very small (a few hundred milligrams).
- The use of some dietary supplements acting on the central nervous system may be potentially harmful to health. A case in point is ephedra, which is found in some herbal supplements and is reported to be used widely in some sports. Ephedra is a stimulant that increases the amount of dopamine within the brain. A number of deaths (from heat illness occurring during exercise) have been either directly or indirectly linked to this supplement. Its use will result in a positive doping test under current WADA rules.

Chapter 19

Weight management

Asker Jeukendrup

Weight loss or weight gain

Weight management is one of the key issues in sports nutrition both for athletes who want to gain weight (muscle mass), as well as athletes who want to lose weight (body fat). This chapter will focus mainly on weight loss, while issues of weight gain are to some degree covered in Chapter 9 "Building Muscle". Weight loss can sometimes be an advantage because it increases the power to weight ratio (in jumping, for example) or because it reduces the energy needed to carry one's body weight (in running, for example). Lastly, some desire to lose weight for aesthetic reasons. Weight loss may not always be a good idea and can even be detrimental to performance.

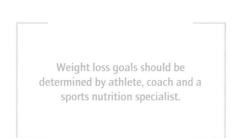

Weight loss goals should be determined by athlete, coach and a sports nutrition specialist.

Where to start

The first step of any weight loss program is to define weight loss goals. These goals should be carefully considered and defined. Is it really desirable to lose body weight? Weight loss may be useful in some cases, but in others it will do more harm than good. Whether it is a good idea or not depends primarily on the body fat percentage. Although individual differences exist, it is not recommended to go below a body fat percentage of about 5% for men and 12-14% for women. Fat has important bodily functions and these will be compromised at extremely low fat levels. The goals also have to be defined with a time table in mind. How much weight do you need to lose and how much time is there to achieve this? A realistic weight loss is about a kilogram every two weeks, so at least 6 weeks are needed to lose 3 kilograms. A more rapid weight loss will make it impossible to train adequately. Weight loss goals should be determined by the athlete, coach and a sports nutrition specialist.

Methods

When the energy intake equals the energy expenditure you will be in energy balance. When you eat less than you burn, you are in negative energy balance and as a result you will lose weight. When you eat more than you expend, you are in positive energy balance—and in this case you will gain weight. A negative energy balance is necessary to lose weight and there are three ways to induce a negative energy balance:

1. Reducing energy intake
2. Increasing energy expenditure
3. A combination of 1. and 2.

Reducing energy intake to lose weight

The most important factor is the reduction in energy intake, although the macronutrient composition of the diet may also have an effect. This has resulted in the often quoted statement a "calorie is not a calorie." Epidemiological studies have shown that both energy restriction and low-fat eating results in weight loss. Energy restriction usually results in a larger reduction in energy intake than does ad libitum low-fat eating. High protein diets have also been shown to be effective. (See the next chapter.)

> Not only energy intake is important, the macronutrient composition of the diet may play a role as well.

Energy restriction may initially result in a larger weight loss, although studies show that both diets are effective over the long term. Reducing dietary fat intake can be a very effective way to reduce energy intake and promote weight loss for several reasons:

- Fat is very energy dense. It has more than twice the amount of energy as the same weight of carbohydrate or protein.
- High-fat foods generally taste good, which leads to a tendency to eat more. Studies show that increasing the fat content of the diet increases the spontaneous intake of food.
- A large body of evidence has also shown that fat is less satiating than either protein or carbohydrate (see Chapter 20).
- Fat is efficiently stored and requires very little energy for digestion.
- Fat intake does not immediately increase fat oxidation.
- Increasing the protein intake can be beneficial as it may help to maintain muscle mass (see Chapter 20) and may increase satiety. However, if the performance of athletes has to be maintained it is important to avoid critically low carbohydrate intakes. What critically low is will depend on the sport, discipline and duration and intensity of the exercise sessions. It also becomes important to carefully monitor fatigue symptoms in these situations. In Chapter 28 examples of questionnaires are provided that can be used to monitor fatigue and prevent overreaching.

Increasing energy expenditure to lose weight

Most athletes can include exercise sessions with the specific aim of increasing energy expenditure, and they can exercise at a high enough intensity to significantly increase energy expenditure. In some sports, however, this often leads to clashes with coaches. For example, coaches of athletes who compete in explosive events (e.g. sprints and jumps) are often reluctant to include aerobic exercise in their training programs. Athletes may also have difficulty finding more time to exercise without compromising recovery from their normal training. In general, however, it should be possible to increase energy expenditure to help weight loss. Important questions then become: what is the best type of exercise? what is the best exercise intensity? and what is the optimal duration? These questions are more difficult to answer. The research is equivocal with regard to the effects of different exercise intensities. Walking and running have been shown to result in higher fat oxidation rates (see Chapter 6), but whether this would result in greater weight loss is questionable. It seems obvious though that a longer bout of exercise and a moderate intensity will increase energy expenditure the most. However, others have argued that, energy expenditure may be elevated in the post-exercise period and that this effect is greater than the effect of the exercise itself. It is well-established that immediately after exercise, EPOC (post exercise oxygen consumption) may be elevated, although this may only occur if the exercise is long and vigorous enough. Even if this is the case, the post exercise increase in resting metabolic rate (RMR) seems only temporary and relatively small. After several hours the RMR will return back to baseline values. Suggestions that resting metabolic rate is chronically increased have been refuted and even though some studies have reported an increased resting metabolic rate, several other studies have even observed a decrease in resting metabolic rate after training.

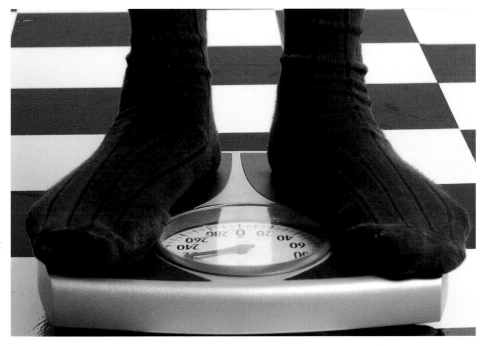

© fotolia, Steve Pepple

The combined approach

A combination of increasing energy expenditure and decreasing intake seems to be the best method for long term body weight loss. Besides In order to lose body fat you need both a negative energy balance and a negative fat balance.. This generally means reducing the fat intake, but including aerobic work in training sessions is another way of moving to a negative fat balance.

Other considerations

There are many supplements on the market with claims to increase fat metabolism and help weight loss. However, these supplements have either no evidence base or have very small effects in comparison to manipulations of macronutrient intake. Some of these supplements, like caffeine, for example, may act on increasing energy expenditure but the effects are small and probably insignificant, especially compared with what can be achieved by exercise and reducing energy intake.

Initial weight loss is usually rapid, but this is mainly because of water losses as glycogen stores are reduced. The loss of body fat will occur relatively slowly.

Another approach that athletes have tried in the past is not eating in the morning and sometimes even skipping lunch. This is not advised because it will increase hunger feelings later in the day; with one single very large meal, the reduction in intake can easily be compensated.

When losing body weight, there is always the risk of losing some muscle mass also. However, this can partly be prevented by consuming relatively large amounts of carbohydrate. Because it is difficult to train hard when the energy intake is reduced, it is advised to achieve weight loss during the off season.

Finally, the loss of body water often accompanies diet-induced weight loss. However, dehydration, losing too much water, can be detrimental to performance. In the end, any athlete should consider the pros and cons of intentional weight loss and should pay attention to unintended weight loss, as this may be a sign of more serious underlying problems.

Energy density

The energy density of the diet plays an important role in weigh management. Interestingly, a number of studies have shown that subjects tend to eat a similar weight of food regardless of the macronutrient composition. Since a 500 gram meal consisting mainly of carbohydrate will contain significantly less energy than a 500 gram high fat meal, this will automatically result in a lower energy intake. Further, visual cues may help prevent a large intake of carbohydrates, which are of high bulk and volume, whereas these cues may not be triggered when regarding a small quantity of fat-rich food which has a very high (relative) energy content.

In an elegant series of studies Stubbs et al. (1995ab, 1996) demonstrated that when subjects received a diet that contained 20%, 40% or 60% fat and could eat ad libitum, the weight of the food they consumed was the same. Thus, due to differences in energy density, the total amount of energy consumed was greater (and weight was gained) with the higher fat diets. This happened both in controlled laboratory conditions as well as in free living conditions. When the fat content of the diet was altered and the energy density was kept the same, the subjects still consumed the same weight of food, but this time the energy intake was independent of the fat content of the diet.

> A number of studies have shown that people tend to eat a similar weight of food regardless of its macronutrient composition and energy content.

Dietary changes to avoid energy dense foods and to include more bulky, low energy dense foods may be one of the keys to success when attempting to lose weight.

Conclusion

Weight loss can be achieved by reducing intake, increasing energy expenditure or both. Weight loss has to be carefully planned by the athlete, coach and a sports nutrition professional. Goals have to be realistic and achievable. There are no shortcuts and there is no substantial evidence that the use of nutrition supplements can result in significant weight loss. Therefore, the athlete will have to balance intake and expenditure giving attention to the macronutrient composition and energy density of the foods. For athletes who want to lose weight while continuing to train, recovery needs special attention and carbohydrate (and protein) intake post- exercise will play an even more important role.

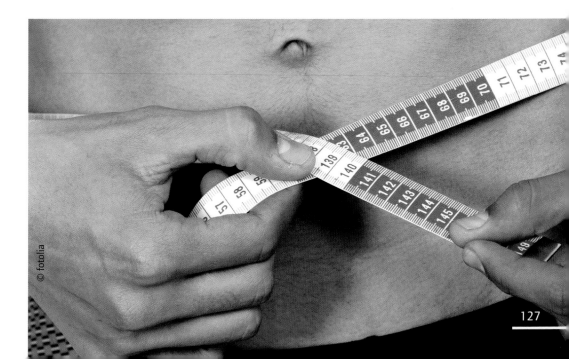

© fotolia

Table 1: Weight loss tips

- Determine a realistic target weight/goal with the help of a sports dietician.

- Do not try to lose more than half a kilogram per week and do not restrict energy intake by more than 500-750 kcal per day.

- Eat more fruit and vegetables.

- Try to choose low-fat snacks.

- Study food labels and try to find substitutes for high-fat foods. Do not only look at fat content but also the energy content per serving.

- Limit fat add-ons such as sauces, sour cream and high-fat salad dressings or choose the low-fat versions of these products.

- Try to structure your eating into 5 or six smaller meals.

- Avoid eating very large meals.

- Make sure carbohydrate intake is high and consume carbohydrates immediately after training.

- Reduce the intake of fats and increase the intake of protein a little.

- Increase the volume of aerobic training to promote fat oxidation. Ideally this exercise should be performed daily for at least one hour at a fairly intensity: it should not be so hard that talking is a problem.

- A multivitamin and mineral supplement may be useful during periods of energy restriction. You should seek the advice of a nutritionist or dietician.

- Measure body weight daily and get measurements of body fat regularly (every 2 months). Keep a record of the changes

Many of these guidelines need specific nutrition knowledge and, therefore, athletes are encouraged to seek the advice of qualified registered sports dieticians.

Chapter 20

Protein and weight loss

Samuel Mettler and Kevin Tipton

Weight control is a significant issue for many people, including athletes. Athletes may want to lose weight for aesthetic reasons or to attain a better power to mass ratio to improve performance. In general, weight loss is accomplished by creating a negative energy balance for a sufficient period of time (see Chapter 19). Thus, decreased energy intake through dietary energy restriction and/or increased energy output through increased activity are necessary. For sedentary individuals, the best strategy likely is to decrease energy intake and increase exercise and habitual activity to lose weight over a relatively prolonged time period. However, many athletes may desire rapid weight loss for competitive reasons and often cannot increase activity levels to any significant degree. Thus, control of dietary energy intake is crucial. Recently, it has become evident that weight loss may be influenced, not only by the total energy intake, but also by the composition of the diet. In particular, protein intake has received a great deal of attention with regard to weight loss.

Weight loss and the influence of protein

A low energy intake relative to energy expenditure is a prerequisite for a negative energy balance and loss of body weight. However, a negative energy balance does not only result in loss of body fat, but also muscle mass, which represents the largest part of lean body mass.

Recently, many studies have demonstrated that increased protein content of the diet, particularly in combination with exercise training, may improve weight loss and reduce the loss of lean body mass in overweight and obese individuals during low energy dieting (Layman et al. 2005). Furthermore, weight regain after the low calorie period ends is less when protein intake is high compared to more normal dietary compositions. Thus, high protein intake seems to be quite advisable during weight loss, at least in obese and overweight individuals.

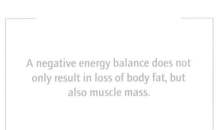

A negative energy balance does not only result in loss of body fat, but also muscle mass.

What is a high protein diet?

Before we recommend a "high protein" diet we have to define what, exactly, is meant by a right protein diet. It is important to differentiate whether the absolute or relative amount of protein is being considered. As indicated in Table 1, the absolute and relative protein content of a diet varies considerably depending on the energy level, which may easily range from 2000 to over 5000 kcal·day^{-1} for different athletes. It is obvious that cutting a small percentage of the energy results in a relative large absolute energy deficit at a high energy level. At the higher energy levels, protein can easily be kept at a high absolute level. On the other hand, athletes with a low energy budget need to increase the relative protein content of the diet much more to maintain or achieve even a moderate absolute protein supply.

Table 1: Comparison of different energy restrictions and the concomitant impact on the relative and absolute protein intake.

	Body mass		Energy	Restriction	Protein		
Elite athlete	80 kg	Normal	5000 kcal		15%	187 g	2.3 g·kg^{-1}
		Weight loss	4000 kcal	20%	15%	150 g	1.9 g·kg^{-1}
		Weight loss	3000 kcal	40%	25%	187 g	2.3 g·kg^{-1}
Male athlete	75 kg	Normal	3500 kcal		15%	131 g	1.8 g·kg^{-1}
		Weight loss	2100 kcal	40%	15%	79 g	1.1 g·kg^{-1}
		Weight loss	2100 kcal	40%	30%	158 g	2.1 g·kg^{-1}
Female athlete	60 kg	Normal	2300 kcal		15%	86 g	1.4 g·kg^{-1}
		Weight loss	1380 kcal	40%	15%	52 g	0.9 g·kg^{-1}
		Weight loss	1380 kcal	40%	30%	104 g	1.7 g·kg^{-1}
Sedentary obese	85 kg	Normal	2000 kcal		15%	75 g	0.9 g·kg^{-1}
		Weight loss	1600 kcal	20%	15%	60 g	0.7 g·kg^{-1}
		Weight loss	1200 kcal	40%	30%	90 g	1.1 g·kg^{-1}

Another question is, whether protein should be increased at the expense of carbohydrates or fat. There is no evidence that the carbohydrate to fat ratio would influence protein requirements. However, the total carbohydrate intake may be crucial for maintenance of proper training, particularly in physically demanding sports. Thus, because an energy cut-off affects the carbohydrate supply per se, an exchange of carbohydrates for protein should be avoided in order to maintain training quality. Consequently, increased dietary protein should be balanced with decreased carbohydrates and fat or fat alone. The energy budget of the athlete as well as individual aspects of dietary and training requirements should be considered.

Protein during weight loss in athletes

In contrast to obese subjects, there are only few data available about the influence of protein on body composition and performance in lean persons or athletes. We recently performed a weight loss study with healthy, young resistance-trained male athletes. They consumed a weight loss diet providing either 15% (1.0 g·kg^{-1}·day^{-1}) protein in the control group or 35% (2.3 g·kg^{-1}·day^{-1}) protein in the high protein group for two weeks. Total weight loss was significantly greater in the control group compared to the high protein group. Interestingly, the weight loss stemmed primarily from a significantly greater lean body mass loss in the control group, whereas fat loss was fairly similar for both groups. This outcome differed from results from studies on obese individuals in several ways. Reduced lean body mass loss also has been shown in obese subjects, but the effect seemed to be more pronounced in the athletes. Further, in obese subjects an increased total body mass loss with higher protein intake often was achieved primarily due to increased fat loss. We found reduced total body mass loss with increased protein largely because of a reduced lean body mass loss. Notably, fat loss has always been much larger than lean body mass loss in obese subjects. In contrast, lean body mass losses exceeded fat losses in our lean athletes at the lower level of protein intake. Other data from studies of athletes also indicate that lean body mass losses may exceed fat losses (Walberg et al. 1988; Mourier et al. 1997), and that lean body mass losses might be reduced with an increased protein content of the diet.

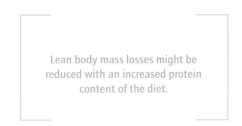

Lean body mass losses might be reduced with an increased protein content of the diet.

The reason that obese and lean athletic individuals respond differently to high protein, low energy diets is unknown. A possible explanation may be found in the influence of body fatness on body composition during weight loss (Forbes 2000). There is evidence that fat is lost in proportion to total body fat at the beginning of the diet period and vice versa. Interestingly, this principel is not restricted to humans; many species exhibit this characteristic.

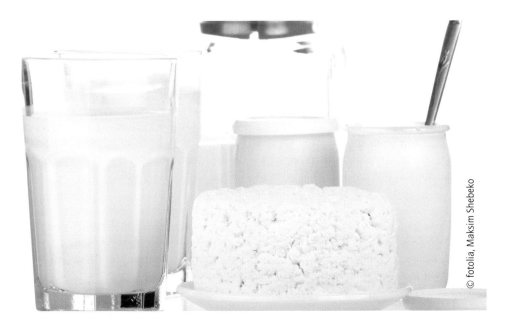

© fotolia, Maksim Shebeko

Dose response

Since we have only begun to investigate the impact of high protein diets on the composition of body weight loss in athletes, it is difficult to define the minimal or optimal protein level for the maximal effect on lean body mass maintenance in athletes. Available data seem to indicate that relatively high amounts of protein, potentially around or even above 2.0 $g \cdot kg^{-1} \cdot day^{-1}$, might be needed to optimally preserve lean body mass in a weight loss situation in athletes. However, further research is needed to determine the optimal level of protein.

Although increased protein intake seems to preserve muscle mass in a situation of negative energy balance, the mechanisms are still not completely understood.

Why protein may preserve muscle

How protein may assist weight loss

In addition to the effect of protein on protein synthesis and body composition during weight loss in laboratory controlled studies, there are other ways that protein facilitates weight loss.

- **Satiety:** There is good evidence that protein has a sustained satiating effect. In other words, the feeling of fullness and satisfaction is increased with increased protein intake. This effect may be particularly helpful in free-living situations, rather than controlled experiments, because it will reduce the motivation to drop out of a low calorie diet.

- **Energy Expenditure:** The loss of body mass, particularly lean body mass, is associated with a reduction in resting metabolic rate (RMR). This reduction means that less calories will be burned, thus potentially compromising the ability to meet weight loss goals. However, RMR is also slowed down by the energy restriction per se. Increased protein may attenuate declines in trijodothyronin, an important hormone for maintenance of metabolic rate, thus maintaining RMR during weight loss.

- **Thermic effect of food:** Protein consumption results in greater energy expenditure following a meal, i.e. the thermic effect of food (TEF), than other nutrients. This increase is due to the relatively large amount of energy needed for the metabolic processing of protein. Therefore, the energy ingested in the form of protein may be considered as metabolically less efficient compared to carbohydrates and fat. Whereas the energy available from protein is the same as carbohydrates, it takes about 25% of that energy to process the protein reducing the net energy gained from eating the protein. Since protein synthesis is energetically expensive, stimulation of protein synthesis by the protein also may contribute to increased energy expenditure.

- **Increased Muscle Protein Synthesis:** Protein and amino acids may stimulate protein synthesis, resulting in an improved net protein balance. This effect of protein seems to be largely attributable to the changes in the levels of essential amino acids, particularly the amino acid leucine. Leucine is a key stimulator of the molecular pathways that initiate protein synthesis. Additionally, extra dietary protein provides amino acid as substrates for protein synthesis – an important consideration since these amino acids will serve as the building blocks for increased muscle.

Summary

The goals of the athlete should be carefully considered before deciding on the appropriate nutritional strategy for weight loss. It seems that increased protein intake may protect lean body mass when a low calorie weight loss diet is implemented. If total weight lost is important, without consideration of what kind of tissue is lost, then a high protein dietary composition may not be desirable. However, if maintaining muscle is crucial, then perhaps a high protein diet would be preferred.

Practical implications

- The protein level of the diet may significantly influence the amount of lean body mass lost during weight loss in lean athletes.

- If the primary goal of an athlete is maximal weight loss, the protein should be kept low (i.e., below 1.0-1.2 $g \cdot kg^{-1} \cdot day^{-1}$) in order to lose body fat and significant amounts of muscle mass.

- If the primary goal of an athlete is to maintain muscle mass as much as possible in order to optimize body composition while losing weight, the absolute protein supply should be kept high, possibly around or even above 2.0 $g \cdot kg^{-1} \cdot day^{-1}$.

- The larger the energy deficit the more lean body mass is lost. Extreme energy restrictions are detrimental for muscles.

- Protein and exercise have additional effects on lean body mass maintenance in obese subjects. In athletes, an additional exercise intervention is often not feasible. Increased training combined with an energy deficit may put athletes at high risk of overtraining. If possible, however, an exercise-induced energy deficit may be less detrimental for muscle mass than a diet-induced energy deficit.

- The higher the energy requirement of an athlete is, the easier it is to maintain protein at a high level (i.e., around 2.0 $g \cdot kg^{-1} \cdot day^{-1}$). Athletes with a low energy budget need to increase the relative protein intake substantially (i.e., >30% energy) in order to attain at least a moderate absolute protein supply.

- Most athletes should not restrict carbohydrate in order to increase protein intake.

Table 2:

Examples of foods high in protein relative to the carbohydrate and fat content.

- A range of lean meat and meat products (e.g. chicken, ham, ostrich)
- Fish (e.g. tuna, codfish, trout, redfish)
- Low fat dairy products (some may be high in sugar)
- Legumes (baked beans, beans and peas)
- Tofu or other meat replacement products
- Sports food may assist timed protein supply and allow more food variety.

© fotolia, Sergey Lavrentev

Chapter 21

Nutrition- and exercise-associated gastrointestinal problems

Beate Pfeiffer

Gastrointestinal (GI) problems are a common concern of athletes especially those competing in prolonged endurance exercise events. In most studies, the incidence of GI symptoms, have been documented as being between 30-50%. Ultimately these symptoms can impair performance and possibly prevent athletes from

> 30-50% of people may report gastrointestinal discomfort during endurance exercise.

performing well or even finishing a race. The causes of GI problems during exercise are diverse, but can be related to the intake of foods before and during exercise. Inappropriate food and fluid intake or foods to which the athlete is unaccustomed can cause GI distress. It is, therefore, vital for athletes to carefully select and test their food and fluid intakes before race day.

It has been demonstrated that exercise at high intensities leads to a redistribution of blood flow such that the priority becomes to nourish the exercising muscle. This may lead to a reduced blood flow into the gut. It has been suggested that this can lead to the development of GI symptoms alongside changes in increases in sympathetic nervous system activity and altered hormonal responses during exercise. The exact causes of GI symptoms, however, are incompletely understood. On top of these exercise induced GI problems; race nutrition can exaggerate or cause a number of GI problems.

What are common symptoms during exercise?

A variety of different GI symptoms can occur during exercise (see Table 1). The reported prevalence of these symptoms varies in different studies depending on the method of investigation, study population, sex, age and training status of the athletes as well as mode and intensity of the exercise studied. Typically a prevalence of 30-50% is reported.

Table 1: Common symptoms during exercise

Upper abdominal problems	Lower abdominal problems
Reflux/Heartburn	Intestinal / lower abdominal cramps
Belching	Side ache / stitch
Bloating	Flatulence
Stomach pain / cramps	Urge to defecate
Vomiting	Diarrhea
Nausea	Intestinal Bleeding

Who is likely to get GI problems?

The prevalence of GI problems varies between different individuals. Generally, females are more likely to experience GI distress than males. This is especially true during menstruation when women tend to experience more gastrointestinal distress. Younger athletes appear to be more susceptible to GI problems than older athletes, which might be due to increased years of training as well as a better experience in terms of the right feeding strategy in the older athletes. It is also known that training status is negatively correlated with the incidence of GI distress.

Aside from "risk factors", there appears to be an individual sensitivity which predisposes athletes to certain conditions. In a set of recent studies the tolerance to different carbohydrate gel intakes during intense running was investigated. A consistent finding was a strong correlation between a history of GI distress and the reported GI symptoms during the trials. This suggests that an individual predisposition to GI problems during exercise exists (Pfeiffer et al. 2009).

Gastrointestinal symptoms are more common in running than in cycling and increase with increasing duration and dehydration.

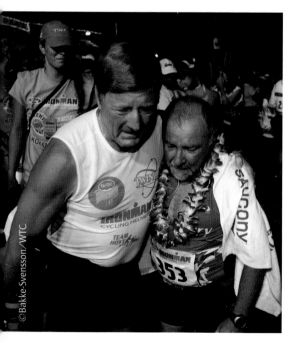

©Bakke-Svensson/WTC

During which sports are GI problems most likely to occur?

The likelihood of someone suffering from GI distress varies between different modes of exercise. GI problems are more common during running than during cycling or any other sport where the body is in a relatively still position such as cross country skiing or swimming. This might be due to increased mechanical stress on the GI tract as a result of the impact experienced with each stride in running.

However, not only the mode of exercise but also the exercise intensity plays a role in the development of GI distress. Lower exercise intensities have no effect on gastric emptying and, if anything, it seems to have a regulating effect on the colon transit. In contrast, high intensity exercise can delay gastric emptying. The blood flow to the gut decreases in proportion to the exercise intensity and GI problems are more likely to occur when the exercise intensity is increased.

Furthermore, a prolonged duration of exercise increases the risk for development of GI distress compared to a short bout of exercise. Toward the end of long races when many athletes become progressively more dehydrated, GI symptoms are more common.

Independent of the sport, race day is always associated with increased psychological stress. Consequently a further attenuation of symptoms through neural and hormonal changes under stress is likely to occur on race day.

Which foods can cause/exaggerate GI problems?

It seems obvious that the athlete has to carefully select foods which are tolerated well and avoid foods that might cause problems (see Table 2).

The digestive process of food in the human body can take about 24 to 72 hours. This suggests that not only the food intake on race day can influence GI comfort but also the nutrition on the days leading up to the race. A high intake of fiber is known to delay gastric emptying of foods, increase intestinal bulk and colonic filling. Therefore, it is not surprising that a relationship has been observed between GI symptoms occurring during exercise and a diet high in fiber. Similarly a diet high in fat is associated with GI distress during exercise possibly due to delayed gastric transit of foods high in fat.

> Food intake on race day as well as the nutrition on the days leading up to the race can influence GI comfort.

It could be hypothesized that the gut is more sensitive during prolonged exercise. If this is the case, mild food allergies and intolerances that are asymptomatic at rest can become an issue during exercise. For example lactose intolerance can be as high as 70% in some populations. Typically one in 10 people is affected. Lactose intolerance is one of the most common food intolerances in many geographical areas. The sensitivity to lactose is caused by a lack of lactase in the gut and the severity of symptoms is dependent on the amount of lactose consumed and the degree of lactase deficiency. It is possible that lactose intolerance is not recognized by an athlete when symptoms during rest are mild. However, there remains the potential that the intolerance can lead to problems during intense exercise when lactose has been ingested.

Table 2: Foods and supplements which may upset the GI tract

Fiber and Fat before and during the race
Hypertonic solutions before and during the race
High carbohydrate intake (in some individuals)
Lactose (if intolerant)
NSAID (e.g. aspirin, acetaminophen (Tylenol), ibuprofen)
Sodium bicarbonate, sodium citrate
High doses of Caffeine
High doses of minerals (e.g. Iron, Magnesium)

Training to drink

In runners, voluntary fluid intake during races seems to be rather small. Dehydration is common and can increase the risk of developing GI distress. On the other hand, it can be a challenge to drink larger amounts during running and the intake of large volumes can also be a cause of GI distress. Interestingly, a recent study showed that the comfortable intake of fluid while running can be increased by training. Runners received a calculated amount of fluid in order to match their sweat loss during repeated training sessions and were asked to rate their GI discomfort. Perceived stomach comfort with a similar amount of fluid ingested was significantly improved in run 5 and 6 compared to the first training session (Lambert et al. 2008).

The choice of drink during exercise has also been associated with the risk of GI symptoms during exercise. Hypertonic drinks have been related to GI discomfort. It is speculated that hypertonic solutions can cause net secretion of fluid into the gut and can lead to abdominal problems such as loose stool and diarrhea. However the degree to which hypertonic carbohydrate drinks can lead to GI symptoms is not conclusive among studies.

In a recent study results showed that large amounts of carbohydrate in the form of gels, delivering up to 90g carbohydrate per hour, had been well tolerated by the majority of runners during a 16km race (Pfeiffer et al. 2009). Nevertheless, in this study a few runners reported severe problems. This leads us to conclude that tolerance of a high carbohydrate intake is different between individuals. The advice for athletes is to test their food and fluid intake during intensive training sessions or during a test race before the actual event.

Other considerations for athletes are possible side effects affecting the GI tract from substances used as supplements or medication. For example, caffeine can have a laxative effect on the GI tract and high doses may lead to GI problems during exercise. Commonly used non-steroidal anti inflammatory drugs (pain killers such as aspirin, acetaminophen and ibuprofen) are linked to GI distress, especially when used in high doses.

What can athletes do to prevent GI problems?

- The occurrence of GI distress is highly individual. Testing of food and drink intake during intense training or less important races is vital.

- Training of fluid intake, especially during running, can reduce discomfort.

- Sufficient fluid intake before and during the race (hydration)

- Avoid fiber rich food (e.g. beans, bran, fruits, and seeded or whole grain bread) intake in the days before the race and during the race.

- Avoid high fat foods in the days before the race and during the race.

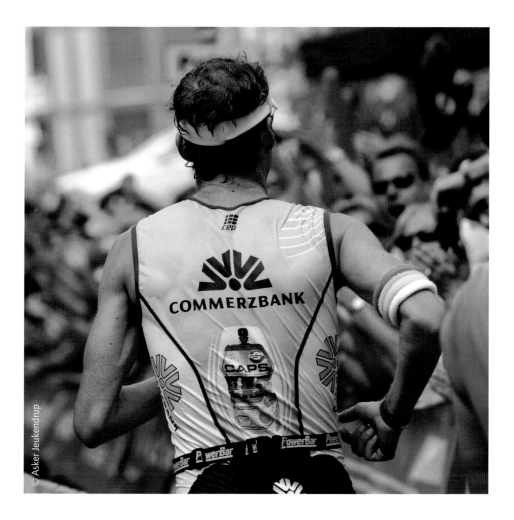

© Asker Jeukendrup

- Allow sufficient time (>3h) to digest the last meal.

- Test your tolerance of lactose and, if sensible, avoid dairy products before the race.

- Caution with NSAID (Non-Steroidal Anti-Inflammatory Drugs): pain killers such as aspirin, acetaminophen and ibuprofen.

- Test use of caffeine before. Possibly reduce dose or split intake into smaller doses

- Test use of sodium bicarbonate or citrate

- Stress management in order to keep psychological stress on race day low

- Adapt intensity to allow normal gut function

Chapter 22

Marathon running

John Hawley

Metabolic demands of the marathon

Many factors contribute to the relative contributions of carbohydrate (CHO) and fat oxidized by the working muscles during marathon training and competition. However, the nutrient and training status of the athlete coupled with the relative running intensity are probably the most important. The process by which skeletal muscle adapts to repeated bouts of exercise over time so that performance capacity is improved is termed physical training. For the competitive marathoner the goal of such training is to increase the pace that can be sustained over a given distance (i.e. 42.2 km). This, in turn, depends on the rate and efficiency at which chemical energy (i.e. CHO, fat and protein) can be converted into mechanical energy for muscle contraction. Therefore, training for marathon racing should aim to induce multiple metabolic and cellular adaptations that enable an athlete to (i) increase the rate of energy production from both aerobic and oxygen-independent pathways; (ii) maintain tighter metabolic control (i.e. match adenosine triphopsphate [ATP] production with ATP hydrolysis); (iii) increase economy of motion; and (v) improve the resistance of the working muscles to fatigue during exercise.

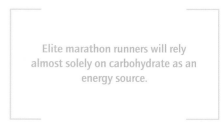

Elite marathon runners will rely almost solely on carbohydrate as an energy source.

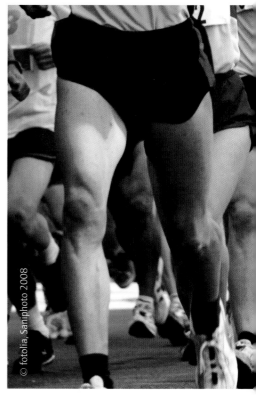

© fotolia, Saniphoto 2008

Elite marathon runners can sustain running speeds equivalent to 80-90% of maximal O_2 uptake (VO_2max) while racing. Recreational runners compete at lower relative intensities. While no direct measurements of the respiratory exchange ratio (RER) have been made during actual competition, it seems possible that elite runners could complete the marathon using only CHO as a fuel. Indeed, studies have shown that for a group of runners who completed a treadmill marathon in 2 h 45 min, the *average* RER was 0.99 (97% of total energy from CHO-based fuels, 3% of total energy from fat-derived fuels) compared to a value of 0.90 (68% of total energy from CHO-based fuels, 32% from fat-based fuels) for slower runners who finished in 3 h 45 min. Daily dietary requirements for marathon training and racing should probably reflect this fuel mix.

Nutritional requirements for marathon training

Several investigations have examined the impact of daily CHO intake on training capacity and subsequent performance in runners. A limitation of these studies is that they typically employ short (up to 2 wk) intervention periods making it difficult to extrapolate the results to the more prolonged periods of training obviously required for marathon preparation. Nevertheless the data demonstrate that run training and subsequent performance are compromised on diets that do not meet the daily CHO requirements of the trained musculature.

> When runners consumed a diet containing 8.5 g CHO·kg⁻¹·day⁻¹ it resulted in better maintenance of physical performance and mood state over the course of a period of intensified training compared with a lower CHO diet (5.4 g CHO/kg BM/day).

For example, a study at the University of Birmingham (UK) determined the effect of two different CHO-containing diets (8.5 versus 5.4 $g \cdot kg^{-1}BM \cdot day^{-1}$) on training capacity, physical performance and mood state during a period of intensified training (Achten et al., 2004). In a randomized cross-over design, seven well-trained runners [maximal O_2 uptake (O_2 max) 64.7 ±2.6 mL·kg⁻¹·min⁻¹] performed two 11-day trials consuming one of the diets. When runners consumed the diet containing 8.5 g·kg⁻¹·day⁻¹ (5% of total energy) it resulted in better mood state over the course of intensified training and maintenance of physical performance (measured by a preloaded 8-km all-out run on the treadmill and 16-km all-out run outdoors), thereby reducing the symptoms of overreaching. While there has been recent scientific interest in how training in the face of low muscle glycogen content might enhance selected nutrient-gene-protein interactions and the cellular signaling pathways central to muscle adaptation, training recommendations based on the limited published data are theoretical, speculative and premature. Accordingly, it seems prudent to adopt recent guidelines for sports nutrition and recommend that the everyday diet of a marathon runner should provide enough CHO to cover the fuel costs of training and restore glycogen content (muscle and liver) between workouts. This is likely to be in the range of 7-10 g·kg⁻¹BM·day⁻¹ according to the volume and intensity of training and the phase of the training program.

> Although there is some evidence that training with low glycogen may result in superior training adaptations there is also evidence that low carbohydrate intake can increase symptoms of overreaching.

Carbohydrate loading and marathon performance

Carbohydrate loading (an increased intake of CHO accompanied by an exercise taper) enhances performance of races lasting > 100 min by enabling runners to sustain goal running pace during the latter stages of a race. While the pioneering studies of muscle glycogen loading employed rigorous diet-exercise regimens to attain supercompensated glycogen levels, a modified version of the diet was developed for trained runners who were able to supercompensate their glycogen stores without such severe demands on their training and CHO status. As such, it is recommended that well trained runners substantially reduce the training volume several days before a marathon race and ensure a CHO intake of 7-10 gCHO·kg^{-1} BM over the final 36-48 h prior to their race.

> Currently the best available monitoring tool for iron status is serum ferritin levels; an individual's history of serum ferritin concentrations is useful to track but intervention is usually undertaken when levels drop below 20 ng/ml.

Carbohydrate ingestion during the marathon

The use of CHO-electrolyte beverages during marathon races is obligatory for most runners. The range of CHO-content (2-10%) provides the runners with the opportunity of manipulating CHO delivery to the working muscles while also altering fluid (i.e., water) intake. The practical issues of fluid and fuel intake depend on the conditions, the sweat rate and personal preferences and tolerance (see also article on triathlon).

Iron status and the marathon runner

Many runners associate feelings of fatigue during training to (undiagnosed) iron deficiency. While iron deficiency anemia is associated with fatigue and impaired exercise performance, and low iron status without anemia interferes with training and recovery. There are many causes of fatigue among athletes and iron deficiency anemia is relatively rare in runners. Low iron status develops when there is an inadequate intake of well-absorbed iron to match iron requirements (increased by growth and pregnancy) and losses (increased by excessive bleeding, blood donation or gastrointestinal blood loss). Iron status should be monitored periodically in runners at high risk of low iron status. Currently the best available monitoring tool is serum ferritin levels; an individual's history of serum ferritin concentrations is useful to track but intervention is usually undertaken when levels drop below 20 ng·mL^{-1}. Intervention to treat iron deficiency anemia or to prevent low iron status from progressing to anemia may include several months of iron supplement therapy. However, this should be followed up by dietary changes to increase the intake of well-absorbed iron, including regular consumption of small amounts of heme iron from animal foods (e.g. red meat, shellfish, liver) and the mixing of foods containing plant sources of iron (e.g. fortified breakfast cereals, nuts and legumes, green leafy vegetables) with foods containing Vitamin C or meat.

Challenges	Solution
Achieving a light and lean physique for optimal performance without going to extremes. Restricting energy intake to below an adequate energy availability can lead to metabolic and hormonal dysfunction.	It is an advantage to be light and lean when carrying your own bodyweight over 42 km. However, each runner needs to find a weight and body fat level that is associated with good health and long-term good performances. A sports dietitian can assist the runner to set appropriate targets and achieve these with sound eating practices.
There is a high prevalence of disordered eating among distance runners, particularly females.	The message to achieve a safe and healthy weight through sound eating practices should be reinforced among marathon runners. Runners who show signs of disordered eating should be referred at an early stage for professional assessment and counseling.
Undertaking key training sessions with appropriate fuelling and hydration strategies	Runners should aim to be well fuelled and hydrated for key training sessions. Daily carbohydrate intake should track the training load to ensure adequate fuelling. Although long runs are often taken in secluded areas, the runner should try to plant drinks and fuel options so that at least some runs are undertaken as a dress rehearsal for race day. Training sessions can be used to get a feel for likely sweat losses, so that an appropriate drinking strategy for race day can be developed and practiced.
Low iron status can interfere with training and recovery; if it further develops into iron deficiency anemia, there is a definite impairment of running performance.	Low iron status can occur in marathon runners because of an inadequate intake of well-absorbed iron to meet iron losses. Runners at high risk of inadequate iron intake (low energy and iron intake and/or increased body iron losses) should monitor their iron status regularly. Treatment of low iron status may involve supplementation with iron while improvements in dietary iron intake and treatment of excessive iron losses are undertaken.
Carbohydrate loading for a marathon requires nutrition knowledge and an appropriate reduction in training volume (i.e., taper).	The runner should reduce their training volume appropriately over the last days prior to the marathon, and follow a diet that provides $10 \text{ g CHO} \cdot \text{kg}^{-1} \text{ BM day}^{-1} \cdot \text{day}$ for the 2-3 days pre-race. Choosing compact, low-fiber fuel-rich foods over the last day of loading should see the runner take the starting line with well-stocked muscle fuel stores and a low risk of gastrointestinal distress.
Choosing a suitable pre-race meal, especially when the marathon starts early in the morning	A light carbohydrate-rich breakfast can be consumed 2-3 hours pre-race according to the previous practices of the runner. Low-fiber, compact choices such as sports bars or liquid meal supplements are often well tolerated.
Achieving appropriate hydration and fuelling during the race to avoid dehydration, hyponatremia or hitting the wall	The marathon usually provides a network of aid-stations that assist the runner to achieve a good race nutrition plan. This plan should aim to replace a reasonable proportion of sweat losses – neither under-drinking to allow dehydration to exceed 2% BM nor drinking excessively large volumes that exceed sweat losses. Practice in training should let the runner develop such a plan. Sports drinks and gels contain carbohydrate and electrolytes to allow other race nutrition goals to be met. A carbohydrate intake of 30-60 g per hour will typically be suitable for additional race fuel needs.

Avoiding gastrointestinal distress during the marathon	Runners who are at risk of GI distress should experiment with avoiding high fiber foods on the day(s) before the race. Other strategies include avoiding concentrated drinks before and during the race. Some runners may need to seek treatment for underlying gastrointestinal problems such as irritable bowel syndrome.
Avoiding muscle cramps during the race	The causes of muscle cramp are largely unknown, are highly individual and may not always be related to nutrition. Some individuals may benefit from magnesium supplementation although evidence is not strong. It must be noted that cramps can be caused by salt imbalances and therefore might also be caused by taking too much.

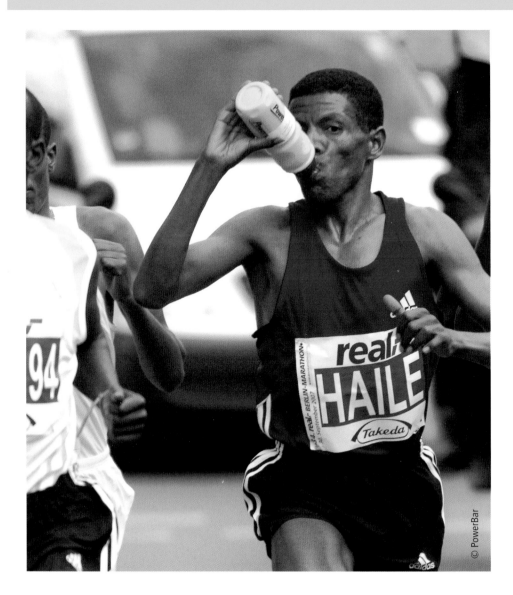

© PowerBar

Chapter 23

Nutrition for middle-distance running

Trent Stellingwerff

Middle-distance racing refers to the events of 800m, 1500m and 3000m, which depending on ability can range in time from 1.5 to 10min However, despite this relatively short race duration, the ATP energy source provision between events and within a given event is incredibly varied. For example, the anaerobic based ATP production (exclusively creatine phosphate (CP) and carbohydrate (CHO) energy) for 800m racing can contribute up to 45% of total energy, while aerobic ATP production (CHO and fat) contributes 88-90% of energy provision for 3000m.

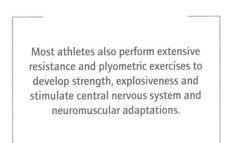

Most athletes also perform extensive resistance and plyometric exercises to develop strength, explosiveness and stimulate central nervous system and neuromuscular adaptations.

Due to this incredible diversity of energy provision between aerobic and anaerobic sources, middle-distance athletes implement a dynamic continuum in training volume, duration and intensity throughout their training year, which utilizes all energy producing pathways (CHO; fat) and muscle fiber types (slow; fast). Furthermore, most athletes also perform extensive resistance and plyometric exercises to develop strength, explosiveness and stimulate central nervous system and neuromuscular adaptations. Accordingly, a middle-distance athlete is probably the most diverse athlete in the athletics arena when it comes to the continuum of required energy provision needed to support a myriad of training stimuli and racing conditions. Middle distance athletes are truly at the cross-roads of metabolism, which is perhaps why many of these athletes can run world-class times in events ranging from 800m to 10,000m. Consequently, a fundamental appreciation of the different fuels (CHO, fat) used during varied training and racing, coupled with the important need for protein (PRO) for repair and recovery of muscle, needs to provide the basis for all acute and seasonal nutritional recommendations.

Periodized nutrition for periodized training

Most middle-distance athletes and coaches tend to structure, or 'periodize', their training throughout the yearly training calendar into phases, with each phase having unique physiological emphasis. There are 4 primary training mesocycles, or phases, that include: 1) general preparation (aerobic/endurance development), 2) specific preparation (anaerobic improvement), 3) competition and 4) rest and recovery (R&R; Figure 1). The stark differences in training volume and intensity between these phases for a middle-distance athlete can be remarkable. An elite middle distance athlete may undertake training during the aerobic development phase that rivals a marathon runners' volume (>150 km·week[-1]; long aerobic runs, threshold training), but during the competition tapering phase training will nearly mimic a long-sprinters' intensity, speed and volume (50km·week[-1]; short runs, sprinting track training). Consequently, the training load and intensity, coupled with the required energy expenditure and fuel selection (CHO vs. FAT) throughout each training phase varies significantly throughout the year, and thus the total and type of nutritional intake should also vary accordingly.

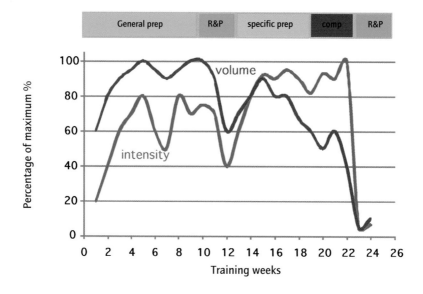

Figure 1: Overview of the major training phases for elite middle-distance athletes.

At the center of this periodized training regime, should be a periodized nutritional approach that takes into account acute and seasonal nutritional needs induced by specific training stimuli (4). As athletes progress through a season of training and racing, from the endurance development phase towards peak championship racing, the relative contribution of CHO derived energy provision increases, while energy from fat sources decreases. Accordingly, dietary CHO ingestion should progressively rise from 55 to 70+% of total energy intake (%En), or 7 to 10 g CHO·kg BW[-1]·day[-1], while dietary fat intake should gradually decrease from 30 to 20% En (1 to 1.5 g FAT·kg BW[-1]·day[-1]), throughout the yearly training plan (1). In terms of daily protein intake, endurance athletes in a hard training phase should ideally consume 1.5 - 1.7 g PRO·kg BW[-1]·day[-1] (5). A non-vegetarian 70 kg athlete consuming 3500 kcal per day would require only about 12% energy intake from protein, which can easily be met in a balanced diet. Finally, it has been shown that ad *libitum* caloric intake is not immediately matched with reduced energy expenditure, as found during tapering in the competition phase.

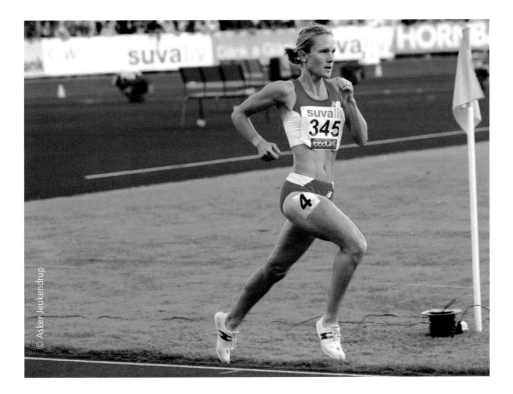

© Asker Jeukendrup

Therefore, athletes need to make conscious decisions about energy intake during this phase, instead of adhering to their habitual diet, to maintain an ideal peak body composition. After the exhausting competition phase and/or training micro-cycle, the athlete must take a period of rest for both mental and physical recovery in which training volume and intensity is generally very low. Due to the diminished, or non-existent, training volume and intensity, nutritional energy intake during this phase/day must be reduced, and thus the macronutrient recommendations are much the same as for the general public (CHO: 4-6 g CHO·kg BW^{-1}·day^{-1}; 0.8-1.2 g·kg BW^{-1}·day^{-1}; 1 to 1.5 g FAT·kg BW^{-1}·day^{-1}). Some weight gain and changes in body composition may occur during this phase, which is natural. However, weight gain should be limited to less than 5% of total BW.

> At the center of this periodized training regime, should be a periodized nutritional approach that takes into account acute and seasonal nutritional needs induced by specific training stimuli.

For coaches and athletes, periodizing the training to peak at the exact time of a major championship is one of the most difficult endeavors to achieve. But, realizing the important and integrated role of nutrition in this quest will bring the athlete one step closer to his or her goals.

Diverse training results in diverse nutritional recovery recommendations

Hard training and racing is catabolic in nature. It is only during recovery, of which nutrition is one of the cornerstones, that the benefits of the hard-work are realized through the recovery of muscle energy stores (primarily glycogen) and the synthesis of new proteins. Most middle-distance athletes utilize an incredibly diverse and varied exercise stimulus. Therefore, depending on the previous exercise mode, intensity and duration, the acute recovery nutritional recommendations will also vary (Table 1).

Table 1: Summary of acute post-exercise dietary recommendations according to specific training type.

Type of Training	Examples of Training Sessions	Fuels Utilized	Acute Nutrition Recommendations
Aerobic capacity & power-oxidative & glycolytic enzymes / VO_{2max} / AT	1) 20 min tempo in 1h run 2) 3x10min on 3min recov. 3) long steady state runs	Mainly FATS	during aerobic training: CHO: 1-1.4 $g \cdot kg^{-1} \cdot h^{-1}$ sports drink exp: 800 to 1000ml sports drink per h
Anaerobic capacity & power-glycolytic enzymes / CHO metabolism / muscular strength / running economy	1) 30 sec reps on 1min recov. 2) 10x1min on 2min recov. 3) hill runs of 15-30sec 4) 90sec reps on 5min recov.	FATS/CHO	short term (<4h) recov: in small repeated doses over first 2h post-exerc CHO: 1.2-1.5 $g \cdot kg^{-1} \cdot h^{-1}$ exp: 800 to 1200ml sports drink per h
		CHO	longer term (>20h) recov: over first 2h post-exerc CHO: 1$g \cdot kg^{-1} \cdot h^{-1}$ total PRO: 0.3 $g \cdot kg^{-1} \cdot h^{-1}$ FAT: 0.1 $g \cdot kg^{-1} \cdot h^{-1}$ exp: 1) whole-wheat bagel + peanut butter 2) 750ml sports drink + protein bar 3) 2 cups cereal + milk + banana 4) tuna on whole wheat + 500ml juice 5) chocolate milk + low-fat fruit yogurt
Explosive training - maximal contraction ability / muscular hypertrophy / technique & economy	1) weight training 2) plyometric jump training 3) sprint & speed drills 4) hill sprints	CHO & ATP/CP	during and 2h post-resistance exerc: CHO: 0.5 $g \cdot kg^{-1} \cdot h^{-1}$ total PRO: 0.3 $g \cdot kg^{-1} \cdot h^{-1}$ EAA: 0.1 $g \cdot kg^{-1} \cdot h^{-1}$ exp: 1) 500ml sports drink + protein bar 2) 250ml of milk + piece of fruit

AT, anaerobic or lactate threshold; CHO, carbohydrate; CP, creatine phosphate; EAA, essential amino acids; exerc, exercise; exp, example; PRO, protein; recov, recovery. (Nutrition recommendations adapted from: 1, 2, and 5).

When the athlete is faced with a short time period for recovery CHO must be supplied immediately to maximize glycogen re-synthesis rates. Contemporary studies suggest utilizing frequent ,smaller doses (i.e. 20-30 g CHO every 20 to 30min) for an overall intake rate of 1.2 to 1.5 g·kg BW^{-1}·h^{-1} for the first several hours of recovery (2). Specifically, this CHO intake protocol is important when an athlete is faced with a short recovery period (<4 h), such as between rounds of races or between hard training sessions on the same day. During these situations, fat should also be avoided as it can slow gastric emptying.

When there is little time in between heats (<4h) it is recommended to eat frequent smaller doses (i.e. 20-30 g CHO every 20 to 30min) for an overall intake rate of 1.2 to 1.5 g·kg BW-1·h^{-1} for the first several hours of recovery.

During longer-term recovery (24 h+) and recovery from resistance exercise, PRO intake in conjunction with CHO is vital to maximize muscle glycogen re-synthesis, protein synthesis rates and the repair of damaged muscle tissues. However, it remains to be clarified what the most ideal macronutrient blend is. What feeding pattern, type of CHO and/or protein (whole intact proteins vs. hydrolyzed) and intake timing optimize recovery and adaptation after different types of exercise stimuli?

Nutrition for travel & competition

The incredible physical strain of competition on a middle distance athlete is made even more arduous with added demands such as intense travel and race schedules, as well as major championship competitions with multiple rounds of racing. For example, during a typical international indoor and outdoor racing season elite male and female middle distance athletes race an average of 18 times per year with 77% of those races being located in Europe/Russia, 17% in Australia/Asia/Africa and 6% in North America (competition year of 2006). Travel is a necessity for the international (level) runner; athletes must compete in major meetings in different countries, each featuring different travel demands, time zones, cultures and climates. With these constraints, athletes are challenged to find appropriate nutrition and hydration for racing, as well as familiar and healthy foods for their general diets.

The task of recovery between rounds at a major championship can be challenging, as middle distance athletes are faced with multiple races, each of considerable energy demand. As an example, Sebastian Coe raced 7 times in 9 days during his 800m and 1,500m double at the 1984 Los Angeles Olympics, which culminated in Olympic silver and gold medals, respectively. Accordingly, a well-practiced competition nutritional regime needs to be established. Some suggestions are outlined below:

- Find several individualized pre-competition meal options that are convenient, readily available, and feel 'right' for the athlete that are high in CHO (1 to 4 g·kg BW^{-1}) and consumed 1 to 6 h prior to competition according to individual preferences.
- Athletes should aim for 400-600 ml of either sports drink and/or water in the 1 to 3h before competition, and many athlete combine this with a small snack (e.g. sports bar, fruit).

- It is vital that the athlete has post-race foods and fluids immediately available, due to the common travel time constraints from the competition site to accommodation location. CHO rich foods and fluids with a medium to high glycemic index at an intake rate of about 1 g CHO·kg BW^{-1}, and 0.3g·kg BW^{-1} should be the target. (See Table 1 for practical examples.)
- Specialized sports nutrition products (carbohydrate-protein energy bars or drinks) can provide many of these initial CHO and PRO needs, and are convenient and familiar, until a normal meal can be consumed.
- All nutrition for competition routines should be practiced and individualized in prior training and lower-importance racing situations.

Supplements and middle distance running

Anaerobic glycolysis provides the majority of energy for middle-distance racing, but results in metabolic acidosis via augmented hydrogen ion (H$^+$) accumulation in conjunction with lactate (La-) production. This augmented H$^+$ accumulation causes a drop in intramuscular pH, which leads to fatigue during high-intensity exercise situations. Potentially, both intra- and extra-muscular buffering of H$^+$ should lead to an increase in performance where metabolic acidosis is a limiting factor. In line with this, supplementation of beta-alanine (β-alanine) and sodium bicarbonate (NaHCO$_3$) or sodium citrate has been shown to augment intra- and extracellular buffering capacities, which may lead to a small, but significant, increase in performance.

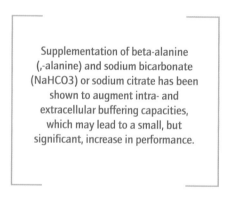

Supplementation of beta-alanine (,-alanine) and sodium bicarbonate (NaHCO3) or sodium citrate has been shown to augment intra- and extracellular buffering capacities, which may lead to a small, but significant, increase in performance.

Several previous studies have directly examined the effects of NaHCO$_3$ ingestion as it applies to middle distance race performance and found ergogenic effects of a 3 to 4 sec improvement in either 800m race time (2:05.8 to 2:02.9) or 1,500m race time (4:18.0 to 4:13.9), respectively. However, consistent and reproducible performance benefits of NaHCO$_3$ loading are not always found, and 50% of subjects experience considerable gastrointestinal- (GI) distress. Thus, data suggests that a given ingestion of 0.3 g of either sodium bicarbonate or citrate·kg BW^{-1}, administered in solution approximately 1 to 2 h prior to exercise ,may offer a small, but significant, effect in middle distance race performance (for review see: McNaughton 2000). The considerable inconsistency between results suggests a high degree of subject variability to dose, performance effect and GI tolerance and, thus, Na HCO$_3$ loading should be well-practiced ahead of time.

Recent evidence has shown that ,-alanine supplementation can lead to an increase in muscle carnosine content, which can potentially result in enhanced intra-muscular H$^+$ buffering, leading to an increase in high-intensity exercise performance. Dosing protocols include taking a single daily dose of 3.2g, or up to 8 daily doses of 0.4 to 1.6g β-alanine per single dose, to reach a total daily ingestion of 3.2 to 6.4 g per day over a range of 4 to 10 wks, which results in a 50-60% increase in muscle carnosine contents. Many studies utilize small repeated doses of β-alanine as it has been documented that large single doses induce mild pseudo-allergic skin reactions of paraesthesia (mild flushing and tingling sensations), that appear to dissipate within several hours. Despite the consistent findings that ,-alanine supplementation leads to an increase in muscle carnosine, the subsequent performance effects have not been so obvious, as about 40% of performance studies have found positive findings. However, of the small number of well-controlled studies showing positive performance outcomes, all have supplemented more than 150g of total ,-alanine over >4 weeks, have shown 40% increases in muscle carnosine (>30 mmol·kg^{-1} dw), if measured, and have used an appropriately controlled anaerobic performance test. It is starting to emerge that when these parameters are accounted for, it appears that b-alanine can significantly improve anaerobic performance. Nevertheless, more well-controlled studies need to be completed to further elucidate the mechanism of action, definitive dosing tolerance/protocols, subject specificity and effects on performance in a range of varying exercise interventions and intensities.

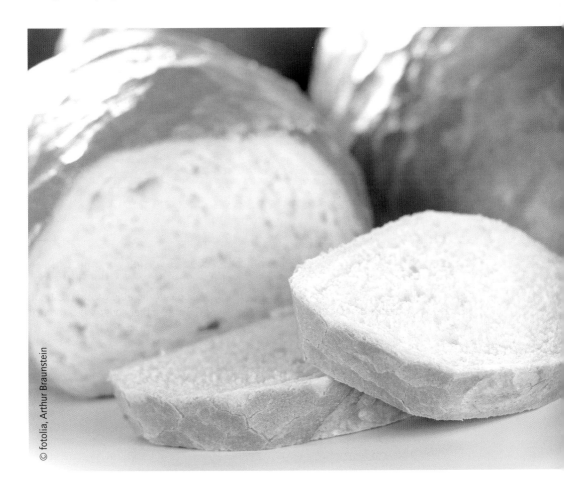

© fotolia, Arthur Braunstein

Chapter 24

Swimming

Louise Burke

Success in pool swimming involves the generation of large power outputs in a highly coordinated and technical manner over races ranging from 20 seconds to 18 minutes. Swimming events are contested in both long-course (50 m pool) and short-course (25 m pool) formats, with long-course swimming being better recognized and included on the Olympic program. Competitions include 1-3 day formats; however, the Olympic (26 events) and World Championship (32 events) programs are typically contested over an 8 day meet of morning and evening sessions (see Table 1). Today, elite swimmers tend to specialize in a few events. Nevertheless, the race programs of exceptional swimmers such as Michael Phelps and Libby Trickett (Lenton) may involve competition on 6 to 7 days of the 8-day program, with two or three races at some sessions (semi-final of one event, final of another event, and a relay leg).

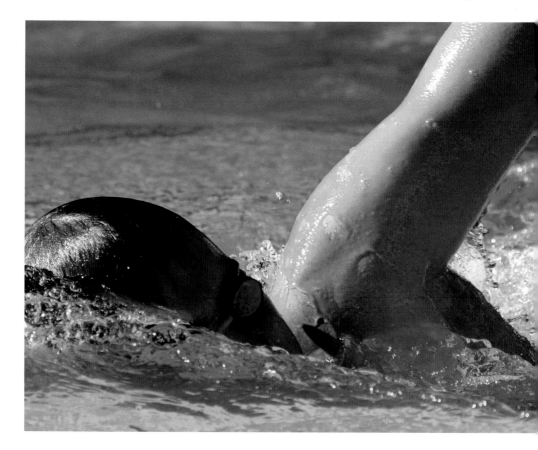

Most elite swimmers undertake a high-volume training program, amassing a total weekly volume of 30-70 km spread over 9 to 12 pool sessions. This is complemented by 3-6 sessions of "dry land" training such as resistance training, flexibility and core strength work, and aerobic activities designed to assist with body composition goals. The training year is divided into phases with weekly microcycles within the longer macrocycles of training, a gradual shift in emphasis from conditioning to race intensity preparation and a defined taper before competition. The consequence is that the nutritional concerns of swimmers involve an amalgam of challenges. During the training phase, swimmers share the priorities of endurance athletes, whereas in the competition setting, the issues are more related to brief duration events. Swimmers begin high volume training at a young age, with exceptional swimmers reaching international standard in their early teenage years.

Nutritional challenges of training

The high training volumes of many swimmers are undertaken against a background of the nutritional issues of adolescence and early adulthood. Early morning training schedules are a ritual of swimming—necessitated by school or work schedules, pool availability, and the desire

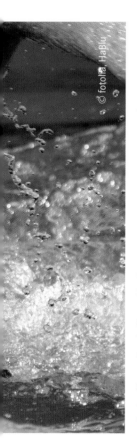

to provide recovery time between the two main workouts in a day. Meals are often eaten on the run, and the family meal schedule often needs to be planned around the training and transport needs of school-age athletes. Many swimmers find it difficult to assume responsibility for their food intake as they move from home to an independent living situation or even the collegiate or institute dining hall.

The developing swimmer often finds conflict between achieving the nutritional goals of their sport while facing the special nutritional, social, and emotional issues of adolescence and early adulthood. In the case of male swimmers, the combination of high energy expenditure in training and the energy needs for growth can lead to exceptionally high requirements for energy and carbohydrate. Many young male swimmers find it difficult to meet such requirements; often suffering from weight loss and fatigue in training. The chief problem for many young female swimmers is coping with the deposition of body fat that occurs during adolescence, particularly during phases of reduced training such as the off-season, taper or injury. Many formerly lean and petite female swimmers struggle with slower performances, poor body image, and battles with their coach over the weight gain and body fat during adolescence. Female swimmers are theoretically at higher risk of developing disordered eating than other athletes because of the need to exhibit their bodies in skimpy clothing. This may be exacerbated by the pressure to conform to the recently observed trend of increased leanness in elite male and female swimmers. Although many swimmers and coaches may see the physique of an elite competitor as the cause of their success, it is difficult to discern the contribution of genetics or the high volume training that resulted in low body fat levels, from the effects of leanness per se. A long-term approach to achieving ideal physique is needed and should encourage each swimmer to find the weight and body fat levels at which they perform well, eat well and enjoy good health. It is important for the swimmer to be able to adjust energy intake according to the volume and intent of their training and racing calendar, and to allow changes in physique within a reasonable range as a result of the differences in these phases. Working with a sports dietitian may help young swimmers to develop the eating practices that will allow them to train well and meet body composition goals now and in the future.

Theoretically, a high intake of carbohydrate is needed to fuel the large volumes of training undertaken by swimmers. Indeed, a classic study by Professor Dave Costill found that swimmers who failed to increase carbohydrate and energy intake when training volume was doubled experienced fatigue and soreness from workouts while the group who spontaneously adjusted their fuel intake were better able to cope with the increased workload. Although inadequate fuel intake for a week didn't impaired subsequent "race" performance, poor nutritional practices might be expected to take their toll when this occurs over a longer period. Dietary surveys of male swimmers typically find self-reported intakes of 15-20 $MJ \cdot day^{-1}$ of energy, providing 6-8 $g \cdot kg \cdot day^{-1}$ of carbohydrate and 1.5-2.0 $g \cdot kg \cdot day^{-1}$ of protein. Allowing for the under-reporting of food consumption that is usually observed in dietary surveys, such intakes seem suitable to meet the nutritional goals of well-trained male swimmers. Dietary surveys and casual observations find that female swimmers typically report energy and carbohydrate intakes that are lower than their male counterparts, and often seem inadequate to support their training volumes. The apparently lower energy and fuel intakes of female swimmers may reflect underreporting, restricted energy intake to achieve fat loss goals, or lower training expenditures. Sports dietitians who work with female swimmers often settle on a plan to periodize energy and carbohydrate intakes, over the week and over the season according to the priorities of body fat/weight goals and fuel needs for training and racing. When energy needs are moderate to large, and a variety of nutritious foods are chosen, most swimmers should be easily able to meet their requirements for vitamins and minerals.

> Studies show that strategies that promote high carbohydrate availability for a training session (carbohydrate intake before and during the workout) can enhance performance of various tasks that might be included in a workout.

A strategic way to meet increased needs for energy, protein and carbohydrate arising from training goals is to plan for the consumption of these nutrients around the workout. This is a useful approach to "periodized eating" for weight/body fat goals in that the swimmers' dietary intake tracks the increases and decreases in training load. However, it may have additional value in promoting optimal training and recovery from each session. Studies show that strategies that promote high carbohydrate availability for a training session (carbohydrate intake before and during the workout) can enhance performance of various tasks that might be included in a workout. In addition, maintaining high carbohydrate availability for workouts might protect the immune system from the decline in function that typically occurs in the hours following a prolonged session of exercise. Staying healthy is a key goal for many swimmers.

The consumption of protein and carbohydrate after resistance training and pool sessions is another example of strategic nutrition to assist in the recovery from, and adaptation to, swimming /workouts. At times of the training calendar many elite swimmers have two or three training sessions scheduled for the day. Quick replacement of these key nutrients after each session will promote refueling and protein synthesis for building new muscle.

Current guidelines based on the available literature recommend a timely intake of 10-20 g of protein and around 1-1.5 g of carbohydrate per kg BM. This may be consumed as a snack eaten soon after the session to promote recovery until the next meal is consumed. In other cases, the swimmer may be able to go straight from training to their next meal and will be able to meet these nutrient targets within the menu. Fluid losses during pool sessions are generally considered to be moderate in comparison to the sweat losses incurred by other athletes or sessions undertaken on "dry land." Nevertheless, it is useful for swimmers to periodically monitor fluid losses over a session or from day to day, particularly in special circumstances such as high volume training in a hot environment or at a high altitude.

> It is useful for swimmers to periodically monitor fluid losses over a session or from day to day, particularly in special circumstances such as high volume training in a hot environment or at altitude.

Of course, it is not always possible or practical for swimmers to achieve high carbohydrate availability for each training session. For convenience, many swimmers will undertake early morning training sessions after an overnight fast or following the intake of very small snacks. It is unlikely that muscle glycogen stores are refueled for each session in a week of high volume training. In fact, the "train low, compete high" hypothesis suggests that some training adaptations might be accentuated when training is undertaken with low glycogen levels. This theory is not yet proven – furthermore, the preliminary support comes from studies in which some, but not all training sessions, were undertaken with low carbohydrate availability. However, it is possible that the best or most practical approach to a heavy training schedule is to promote strategic eating around key training sessions in the program (e.g. sustained high intensity and race-pace sessions, resistance workouts), while allowing a more relaxed approach to fueling up for lower intensity sessions.

Nutritional challenges of racing

Most elite swimmers will peak for important competitions 2-3 times in the year. This involves a substantial taper or reduction in training volume prior to the meet, resulting in reduced energy and fuel requirements. The taper provides an increase in "leisure time" for the swimmer and often occurs simultaneously with a change in the swimmer's environment due to travel for competition. The swimmer needs to follow an appropriate meal plan that meets real energy and fuel requirements for taper and racing, and avoids the distractions/pitfalls associated with eating at athlete dining halls, hotels or host families.

> It is valuable to be self-sufficient by having a supply of foods/snacks at poolside that can promote rapid recovery between or after races. Often it is more practical to rely on special sports foods such as sports bars and ready-to-drink liquid meal supplements.

The fuel requirements for racing are generally lower than those experienced in training. However, swimmers in longer events (400-1500 m) or programs involving several events within the same session should ensure that adequate fueling occurs between sessions, between warm-up and races, and between events. It is valuable to be self-sufficient by having a supply of foods/snacks at poolside that can promote rapid recovery between or after races. Everyday foods such as fruit, sandwiches, cereal bars and flavored yoghurt and milk drinks can supply protein and carbohydrate towards recovery targets. Often it is more practical to rely on special sports foods such as sports bars and ready-to-drink liquid meal supplements. At top levels of competition, the swimmer often faces many distractions after their event which may interfere with their access to food or their ability to eat a substantial meal – these include media commitments, and the requirement to attend doping control to provide a urine sample.

Unless a plan of suitable snacks and quick meals has been organized, the swimmer may find themselves having to sacrifice precious "sleep time" before the next competition session for time to find an opportunity to meet their recovery nutrition goals. A summary of practical ways to address the challenges of training and race nutrition is provided in Table 2.

Supplements and sports foods for swimming

Like all athletes, swimmers are fascinated by the array of sports foods and supplements that promise improved performances. Among the many products on the market, there are a few that offer legitimate benefits to the swimmer – either in helping them reach their nutritional goals, or by directly enhancing performance and recovery. Table 3 provides a summary of these products and their potential uses by swimmers. It should be noted that even when the use of supplements and sports foods can be beneficial, it must be weighed against the expense of products and the potential for negative outcomes. These include poor responses in some individuals, or the risk of a positive doping outcome from contaminated supplements. Such risks can be minimized by trialing products in training, and by choosing products only from well-known companies who have a reputation for strict quality control. Nevertheless, it is generally accepted that the use of ergogenic aids, even when supported by science (e.g. bicarbonate, caffeine, creatine), is not recommended for children (e.g. swimmers under 18 y).

Table 1: Events on the International Program for Swimming

Summary	Events	Times for world class competitors (min:s)
26 events on Olympic program	50 m *Freestyle, backstroke, [a]breaststroke, [a] butterfly[a]	0:21-0:32
32 events on World Championships program	100 *Freestyle, backstroke, breaststroke, butterfly	0:47-0:68
	200 m *Freestyle, backstroke, breaststroke, butterfly, individual medley	1:44-2:26
Events of 50-200 m involve heats, semi-finals and finals	400 m *Freestyle, individual medley	3:40-4:48
	800 m *Freestyle[b]	7:39-8:40
	1,500 m *Freestyle[c]	14:34-17:30
Events of 400-1500 m and relays involve heats and finals	Relays *4 x 100 m freestyle, 4 x 100 m medley, 4 x 200 m freestyle	3:15-8:00

[a]Not on Olympic program; [b]Olympic program only includes this event for women; [c]Olympic program only includes this event for men

Table 2: Challenges and solutions for the swimmer during the training phase

Challenges	Solutions
Achieving and maintaining an ideal weight and body composition	It takes years of training, maturation and healthy eating for a swimmer to attain their ideal physique. Swimmers and their coaches should invest over the long-term to find the weight and body fat level at which the swimmer is healthy, happy and able to perform well. In particular, the swimmer should learn to adjust their food intake to meet changing needs for energy and carbohydrate. Many swimmers gain unnecessary amounts of body fat by overeating during taper, racing and the off-season or injury.
Providing adequate fuel for training	The swimmer should consume carbohydrate according to the fuel needs of their training program. While extra carbohydrate can be consumed with meals during periods of high volume training, it is also useful to organize strategic eating around training sessions. This means having a high-carbohydrate meal prior to sessions, consuming sports drinks or gels during the session and refueling quickly after training. It may not be practical or within the swimmer's energy budget to achieve this for all workouts; however, proactive eating can be focused on the key training sessions of the week.
Recovering between 2-3 training sessions in the day	The speedy availability of key nutrients will promote efficient refueling, adaptation, and rehydration. The swimmer should organize their plan of snacks and meals to provide carbohydrate and protein soon after the key training sessions of the week.
Achieving appropriate energy and fuel intake during a race taper and competition	The swimmer should adjust their intake of food and recovery snacks to meet their reduced needs for energy and fuel. While it is important to be well-fuelled for racing, it is easy to overeat real energy needs.
Facing the most important competitions in a strange environment. "All you can eat" dining, lack of supervision from Mom/home/ coach and the challenges of foreign cuisine are all part of package for high level athletes	The swimmer should identify the challenges of travel including poor access to important foods at the right times, the distractions of "all you can eat" buffets, and food hygiene issues. A pro-active plan includes bringing supplies from home, and being careful to look after individual needs regardless of company or environment. A team plan can support the swimmer to meet their goals.
Recovery between events in a session or between sessions	Many swimmers will compete in a number of races in a single session, or a succession of races culminating in the gold medal. Each swimmer should devise a plan to promote refueling and rehydration between events, which includes consideration of obstacles that will stand in the way of having access to suitable foods at critical times.

Table 3: Sport foods and supplements that are of likely benefit to swimmers

	Product	Comment
Use in achieving documented nutrition goals	Sport drinks	• Used to refuel and rehydrate during prolonged workouts and to rehydrate after the session. Contain some electrolytes to help replace sweat losses and increase voluntary intake of fluid
	Sport gels	• Convenient and compact carbohydrate source for use during prolonged workouts, particularly to refuel when fluid needs are less important
	Sport bars	• Convenient, portable, and easy-to-consume source of carbohydrate, protein, and micronutrients for a pre- or post workout/race snack or to provide additional energy intake over the day
	Liquid meal supplements	• Convenient, portable, and easy-to-consume source of carbohydrate, protein, and micronutrients for post-workout or post-race recovery • Well-tolerated pre-race or pre-workout snack • Low bulk source of energy, fuel and protein especially to support resistance training program or growth
	Multivitamin and mineral supplements	• Supplemental source of micronutrients for the travelling swimmer when food supply is not reliable. • Supplemental source of micronutrients during prolonged periods of energy restriction (female swimmers).
Strong potential for ergogenic benefit	Caffeine	May enhance competition performance when consumed in small-moderate doses (2-3 mg·kg) pre-race, but further studies are needed to investigate the range of swimming events and the range of doses and consumption protocols (e.g., the timing of the prerace caffeine intake) that are effective. Large amounts of caffeine should be avoided since they interfere with sleep and are likely to jeopardize rest and recovery during a multi-day competition program.
	Bicarbonate or citrate loading	The acute use of bicarbonate or citrate to increase blood buffering capacity (e.g., 300 mg·kg BM bicarbonate or 500 mg·kg BM citrate taken 1-2 h prerace) might enhance the performance of 200-800 m swimming events. Alternatively, longer-term loading protocol can be used over a number of days leading up to the competition (e.g., 500 mg·kg·d for 5 days spread into a series of doses over the day) to achieve a more sustained increase in buffering capacity.
	Creatine	Studies show that creatine loading enhances the performance of exercise involving repeated high-intensity work bouts with short recovery intervals. The most likely benefits for swimmers may come from enhancing the outcomes of interval and resistance training. Typical protocols for creatine use: loading dose: 20-30 g in multiple doses (e.g., 4 · 5 g) for 5 days followed by maintenance dose of 2-5 g·day. Uptake appears to be enhanced by consuming creatine with carbohydrate-rich meal or snack.

Chapter 25

Triathlon

Asker Jeukendrup

Triathlon is a sport that combines three disciplines (swimming, cycling, and running) and competitions typically last between 50 min (Sprint distance) and 8-16h (Ironman distance). The causes of fatigue in the short versus the long distance triathlons are different and therefore the nutritional requirements are different. However, in most events dehydration and carbohydrate depletion can be contributing factors to fatigue.

Table 1: Different triathlon events and their typical duration

Event	Typical duration
Sprint distance triathlon	50 – 90 min
Olympic distance triathlon	1h50 – 2h30
Ironman 70.3 distance (or Half Ironman distance)	3h50 – 6h
Ironman or equivalent	8h – 16h

Training nutrition in Ironman, Ironman 70.3 and similar events

Ironman poses a number of nutritional challenges some of which are summarized in Table 2. In an Ironman, participants will expend 8000-11,000 kcal! Also in training energy expenditures can be high. Typically training will require 500-900 kcal per hour depending on the intensity and the fitness level of the athlete. This energy will have to be replenished.

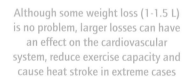

Although some weight loss (1-1.5 L) is no problem, larger losses can have an effect on the cardiovascular system, reduce exercise capacity and cause heat stroke in extreme cases

Since carbohydrate is the main performance fuel, this should be the highest priority. On race day it will be impossible to replenish all the energy but on most training days this should be no problem. As a general guideline, carbohydrate intake should be at least 5 g CHO per kg per day (a 70 kg person would need to take 350 grams of carbohydrates on board). If training becomes longer and harder and more and more glycogen is used, the carbohydrate needs could increase up to 7-8 g·kg·day[-1]. This would apply to people who train 3-4 hours a day for several successive days. In extreme cases even higher carbohydrate intakes would be recommended. Protein requirements are normally around 1 g·kg⁻¹·day⁻¹ and these requirements may increase somewhat with the increased training. However, because athletes eat more anyway to compensate for the increased energy expenditure, protein intake will increase automatically and this is usually not a concern. Fat intake simply makes up for the rest. The 70 kg person, for example, who trains 2 hours per day and expends 3500 kcal per day needs 7 g·kg⁻¹ or 500 g of carbohydrates. This is 2000 kcal. Protein intake would likely be close to 1.2 g·kg⁻¹ or 80 g per day (320 kcal). Fat will make up for the remaining 1180 kcal which is approximately 110 grams. Without performing a detailed nutrition analysis it is difficult to know what this means for your diet, but generally, a bit more focus on carbohydrate and eliminating some fat from the diet will achieve this goal. When the energy intake increases further, there is actually more room for fat in the diet.

High training volumes also have an effect on fluid balance. Sweat rates can vary between 200 mL·h⁻¹ to 3000 mL·h⁻¹! Although some weight loss (1-1.5 L) is no problem, larger losses can have an effect on the cardiovascular system, reduce exercise capacity and cause heat stroke in extreme cases. Therefore, athletes should make sure they drink to prevent large weight losses. In addition, it is wise to check sweat losses on a regular basis simply by measuring (nude) body weight before and after training and correcting for fluid consumption. By doing this regularly you will get a good idea of you sweat losses and this will give you a very good indication of how much you should be drinking. Water is a great drink for hydration purposes but because often you want to fulfill other requirements as well (i.e., energy needs) carbohydrate containing drinks are useful to kill two birds with one stone.

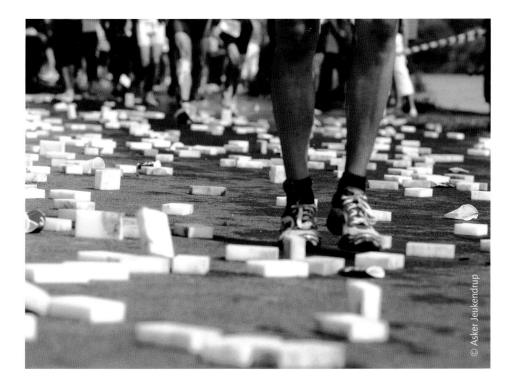

© Asker Jeukendrup

Race nutrition

Most of the carbohydrate and fluid requirements are not very different during training and racing. Adequate carbohydrate stores and hydration before and sufficient supply of carbohydrate and fluids during a race is crucial. However, it must also be noted that very high water intakes may contribute to the development of hyponatremia (low blood sodium).

Salt tablets are normally not needed. However, Ironman races in extreme conditions may be an exception since high salt concentrations (in sweat) combined with high sweat rates, can result in depletion of body salts.

Most commercially available drinks contain sodium, which has been shown to help the water absorption. The salts in these drinks help to replenish salt losses in sweat although in most situations replacing these salts is not all that important. In training there is usually plenty of time afterwards to replenish the salts. Ironman races in extreme conditions may be an exception since high salt concentrations (in sweat) combined with high sweat rates, can result in depletion of body salts. Such high salt losses have been associated with hyponatremia and also anecdotally with the prevalence of muscle cramp. Salt tablets may help in these extreme cases.

The optimal amount of fluid to be consumed during a race is highly individual and can only be determined by regularly measuring body weight before and after training sessions. After a while it is possible to predict a certain weight loss for certain environmental conditions and certain exercise intensities. Once you have worked out your sweat rate it is advised to minimize weight losses and drink fairly close to your sweat losses.

Carbohydrate intake during the race

During any event longer than about 2 h carbohydrate intake can prevent hypoglycemia and improve endurance performance. Ingestion of up to 60-70 g carbohydrate per h has usually been recommended. This recommendation stems from the observation that ingestion of more carbohydrate would not actually result in higher oxidation rates and may accumulate in the intestine.

More recently, however, it was demonstrated that the ingestion of combinations of carbohydrate (glucose +fructose and maltodextrin+fructose) can result in higher oxidation rates, reduced fatigue and better performance when ingested at rates around 90 g•h^{-1}. It is interesting to note that ingestion of glucose and fructose drinks has also been associated with faster

Ingestion of combinations of carbohydrate (glucose+fructose and maltodextrin+fructose) can result in greater fuel delivery, reduced fatigue and better performance when ingested at rates around 90 g/h. These carbohydrate mixtures have also been associated with faster gastric emptying and fluid delivery compared with a glucose drink.

gastric emptying and fluid delivery compared with a glucose drink. The recommendation for Ironman races therefore is to ingest 90 g·h^{-1} of a carbohydrate mixture (See Chapter 4). This can be in the form of a drink, a gel or solid food, depending on personal preference and tolerance.

Tolerance is an important issue as a large number of triathletes will display symptoms of intestinal discomfort during races. These symptoms appear to be related to a number of factors: a high carbohydrate intake or high osmolality drinks ingested during exercise, fiber and fat intake and occasionally milk intake the day or days leading up to a race. When GI symptoms occur during the race, reduce the exercise intensity if necessary. Often this is the only way to control the symptoms. See Chapter 21 for more advice on preventing gastrointestinal distress.

Plan some training rides to practice the nutrition strategy you will use in competition! Use the same products, and the same intake (which is usually higher than what you would do in training) to determine your tolerance to them.

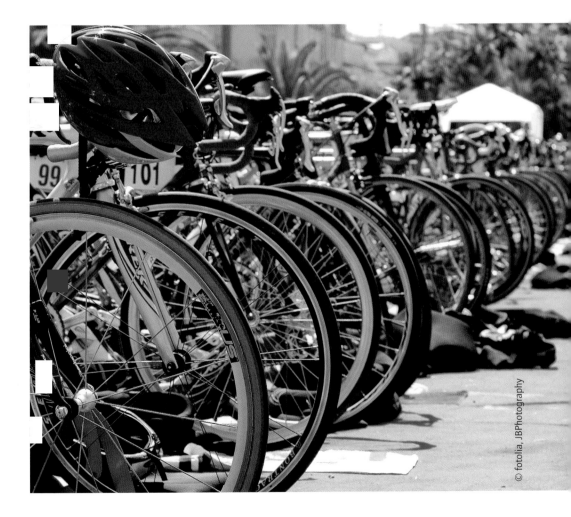

© fotolia, JBPhotography

Table 2: Nutritional challenges and solution for Ironman, Ironman 70.3 and similar events

Challenges	Solutions
Starting adequately fueled and hydrated	Carbohydrate load the days before a race (>7 g·kg⁻¹), (but do not overeat) and drink plenty of fluid
Avoiding running out of energy during the race	Ingest 60-90 g of carbohydrate per hour. When ingesting more than 60 g/h make sure that the carbohydrates are a mixture of glucose and fructose, or maltodextrin and fructose. 90g/h of a mixture (2:1) of glucose and fructose has been shown to improve performance over a single carbohydrate source (glucose). These carbohydrates can be ingested in the form of a drink, a gel or an energy bar or a mixture thereof depending on personal preference and tolerance.
Avoiding dehydration during the race	Obtain an estimate of sweat rate. This can be done by measuring body weight before and after training sessions and correcting for fluid intake. Try to minimize fluid losses to within 2% of body weight.
Avoiding gastrointestinal distress during the race	Avoid high fiber intake in the day (or even days) before a race, avoid high fat intake during the race, avoid drinks with high osmolality, avoid dehydration, reduce the exercise intensity when necessary as often this is the only way to control the symptoms.
Avoiding hyponatremia during the race	Do not drink large volumes of water that exceed the sweat losses. Choose drinks and gels that contain sodium and/or take salt tablets during the race (in moderation).
Avoid muscle cramps during the race	The causes of muscle cramp are largely unknown, are highly individual and may not always be related to nutrition. Some individuals may benefit from magnesium supplementation although evidence is not strong. It must be noted that cramps can be caused by salt imbalances and therefore might also be caused by taking too much.
Consuming enough carbohydrate during periods of hard training	Ensure a high carbohydrate intake and increase with increasing training load.

Sprint distance and Olympic distance

When the distance is shorter and the intensity is higher, some of the above advice still applies. Hydration is still an important issue and carbohydrate intake during the race can still be beneficial. Even in events as short as 1 h carbohydrate ingestion during exercise has been associated with improved performance, although the mechanisms may be completely different. Studies showed that even a mouth rinse with a carbohydrate solution can improve performance during events lasting approximately 1 hour. So even though the participants in this study did not swallow the drink and therefore did not ingest any carbohydrate, the drink still worked. The most likely explanation for this is that carbohydrate binds to receptors in the mouth and this has certain stimulatory effects on the brain (see Chapter 18).

The amount of carbohydrate needed, however, may not be as high as during longer distance races (Table 3).

Table 3: recommended CHO intake during exercise

	Carbohydrate ingestion during exercise		
Sprint triathlon	Very small amounts of CHO	*	*
Olympic distance triathlon	Small amounts of CHO	Up to 30 g·h^{-1}	Can be achieved with most forms of CHO
Half Ironman distance (Ironman 70.3)	Moderate amounts of CHO	Up to 60 g·h^{-1}	Can be achieved with CHO that are rapidly oxidized
Ironman or equivalent	Large amounts of CHO	Up to 90 g·h^{-1}	Can only be achieved by intakes of multiple transportable CHO

Chapter 26

Adventure racing and ultra marathons

Mark Tarnopolsky

Adventure racing is a sport that usually combines three core disciplines (running/trekking, paddling, and cycling) and navigation and can last between 4 hours and 10 days (Table 1). There are often mountaineering skills required including rapelling, ascending, and abseiling. The nutritional recommendations for the shorter adventure races or ultra events are no different than those for the half- and full-Ironman athletes, given that the events are of similar duration and intensity. Under such circumstances, factors such as adequate hydration, carbohydrate availability (exogenous and endogenous), and avoidance of hyponatremia are important and suggestions given in Chapter 25 are applicable.

Only under periods of involuntary (acute altitude) and voluntary (purposeful) energy restriction would an athlete be at risk of consuming inadequate amounts of protein.

There are important issues that emerge when the events approach and exceed 24 h in duration including sleepiness and food avoidance and preference issues. In many of the adventure races and some of the ultra runs, altitude poses a unique challenge due to the anorectic effects of hypoxia. Transportation issues also pose unique challenges to the athletes involved in longer events, especially when the event is unsupported.

Table 1: Examples of ultra-endurance sports and adventure races.

Event (example)	Typical duration
Sprint adventure race, 50 km, 50 mi run	4h – 8h
Overnight adventure race (USARA Championships), 100 mi run (Western States Endurance Run)	16 – 24 h
Multi-day endurance event/stage race (Keen Challenge, Marathon des Sables)	3 – 14 h x 2 + days
Continuous expedition race (Primal Quest)	2 – 10 days

Considerations for the habitual intake of all adventure racers and ultra-event athletes

Given the extreme duration of the events involved, most athletes train a minimum of 2 hours a day and some many more than this. Consequently, it is important to ensure that energy intake is adequate. For most athletes, it is not too difficult to maintain energy balance due to the exquisite regulation of intake to expenditure mediated by the hypothalamus. However, there are several situations in which this balance can be disturbed and athletes tend to consume too few calories. Energy intake always decreases at altitudes over 3000m and the Operation Everest II study clearly showed that this was a function of hypoxia and not reduced food availability. The anorectic effect of altitude would become an issue for example during a training camp at altitude for a lowlander but would not pose an issue for those habitually living at altitude (as a number of top sport ultra athletes do). The maximum daily protein requirements are 1.7 g·kg·d^{-1} and any athlete consuming an energy adequate, balanced diet will get enough protein to meet any increased need. One study found that the mean protein intake for male and female adventure racers was > 1.9 g·kg·d^{-1}. Only under periods of voluntary (purposeful) or involuntary (acute altitude) energy restriction would an athlete be at risk of consuming inadequate amounts of protein.

It is generally recommended that well trained endurance athletes consume > 7 g g·kg^{-1}·d^{-1}. Although most men, and some women, attain this level of habitual intake, a recent study of the habitual intake of adventure racers found that the mean intake for men was only 5.9 g·kg^{-1}·d^{-1}. The latter intake is likely not sufficient for an athlete training over multiple consecutive days, especially if they are doing more than one sport in a day. A carbohydrate intake of 8-10 g·kg^{-1}·d^{-1} is recommended in the 3-4 days before a race to ensure adequate glycogen stores at the start of the race. Although some may argue that glycogen loading before an ultra-event is illogical since the intensity is relatively low (45-65 % of heart rate max on average for a multi-day race), the added water that accompanies the glycogen is of benefit in warm climates and the start of the race is often at a much higher intensity and an early lead can be psychologically as well as strategically advantageous (e.g. first to a rappel or river cross).

Some athletes find that calcium-magnesium (e.g. Rolaids) or calcium carbonate (e.g. Tums) can help to minimize cramps during an adventure race and can have an added benefit of reducing GI upset.

Most athletes consume adequate amounts of vitamins and minerals provided that the diet is balanced, varied and energy sufficient. If any of the above factors are altered, there is a risk of deficiency of a macro- or micro-nutrient. One study in ultramarathon runners found that men and women met the government recommendations for vitamins and minerals, while another study of adventure racers found that some men had inadequate intake of magnesium, zinc and potassium and women had sub-optimal intake of calcium and vitamin E. Women are also at higher risk of iron deficiency due to the menstrual loss and low intake of bio-available iron. Routine iron supplementation is not recommended for women (or men), but an assessment of iron stores is prudent and diet or supplement advice may be needed only if stores are inadequate. Although calcium intake is not performance enhancing, it is important that women consume > 1,000 mg elemental calcium·d^{-1} and vitamin D 1,000 IU·d^{-1} to prevent osteopenia > osteoporosis (especially if amenorrheic or on a low energy diet). Although not supported by the literature, most ultra-athletes consume a variety of vitamin and mineral and anti-oxidant supplements on a daily basis. Conceptually, there does not appear to be any harm in taking a balanced multi-vitamin supplying micronutrients at about the levels recommended by the major governments of the world; however, there may be negative effects from the routine consumption of anti-oxidants during training. Two studies have found that suppression of free radical generation during exercise can attenuate some of the signals for endogenous adaptation.

Table 2: Practical suggestions for the pre-race diet for the ultra-athlete

Nutritional recommendation	Practical tip
Stay hydrated before the race.	• Consume fluids until urine is clear.
Carbohydrate load (8-10 g·kg·d) for 3-4 days before.	• Eat a variety of pastas, breads, fruits, vegetables, cereals.
Consume more sodium and potassium – especially if it is hot and humid for 3-4 days.	• Use a salt shaker, eat fruits and drink fruit juices, eat some salty foods (potato chips, pretzels), pizza (low fat baked crust).
Do not consume too much alcohol if you do drink alcohol.	• Limit intake as a function of experience and probably no more than 2 drinks for men and one for women on the night before a race.
Do not alter the types of foods that you are accustomed to before a race.	• Avoid novel foods in the 3 days before a race. • Stick with what you have tried in the past that did not give you heartburn or flatulence.
If you are a habitual caffeine consumer, do not forget to drink coffee or tea before the race.	• Take in 3-6 mg·kg^{-1} of caffeine about one hour before the start of the race (1 cup coffee 125 mg caffeine; 1 cup tea 50 mg caffeine).
Eat a high carbohydrate/low fiber snack 1-3 hours before the start of the race.	• Try different foods before training and racing to see what is most tolerable for you, examples would include: bagels, toast, fruit, juice, granola bars.

General nutritional strategies before and during an ultra-race

In the 3-4 days before a race it is important to consume > 8 g·kg^{-1}·d^{-1} and to stay well hydrated. Some women may find it difficult to consume > 8 g·kg^{-1}·d^{-1} and may have to increase energy intake during this time. It is particularly important to have a high carbohydrate intake and some protein as soon as possible after finishing a stage in a multi-day race for it could be only a few hours before the next stage and it is important to maximize glycogen re-synthesis. From an energy intake perspective, it is reasonable to plan for at least 400 kcal·h^{-1} for women and 600 kcal·h^{-1} for men. In spite of best practices, most studies do show that adventure racers or multi-sport athletes do lose some weight during a race and there is a clear shift towards oxidizing more of the endogenous lipid stores after a multi-day event. To avoid food aversion (and calorie reduction), it is very important to eat foods that are familiar to the athlete. A new type of food may lead to gastrointestinal upset or reduced food intake due to unpalatability. A major issue when travelling to remote areas or foreign countries is the availability of non-contaminated food and water. If sanitation or availability of food is uncertain, it is important to bring pre-packaged food and drink (or a method of safe sterilization). The consumption of bismuth subsalycilate may work as a prophylactic agent for traveler's diarrhea and it is prudent to discuss anti-biotic use with a physician prior to traveling into an area where diarrheal illness is common.

> From an energy intake perspective, it is reasonable to plan for at least 400 kcal/h for women and 600 kcal/h for men.

Caffeine is very commonly consumed by adventure racers and ultra-endurance athletes. Numerous studies have found an ergogenic effect on endurance exercise performance from caffeine consumption taken in the hour prior to an event at doses as low as 1 mg$\cdot$kg^{-1} to about 6 mg$\cdot$kg^{-1}. For the habitual caffeine consumer, it is very important to have a source of caffeine in races lasting more than 16 hours for most people will undergo withdrawal symptoms at about this time if no caffeine is consumed. The resultant headache and irritability would be particularly troublesome with the added stress of adventure racing with team dynamics and navigation as added stressors. Caffeine intake is common in ultra-events even for those who are not habitual caffeine consumers, due to the well known wakefulness promotion properties that become a major issue when trying to exercise for > 16 hours continuously.

A particular concern for individuals with a low habitual intake of calcium, magnesium and potassium (mentioned above) is the high incidence of muscle cramps that are reported during adventure races and ultra-endurance sports. Although routine supplementation with magnesium during a race has not been conclusively shown to prevent muscle cramps, it is prudent to at least ensure that dietary intake is sufficient to prevent a deficiency situation. Given that muscle cramps during exercise are clearly multi-factorial, it is important to consider that an imbalance of sodium, potassium, calcium or magnesium may be a factor. Some athletes find that calcium-magnesium (e.g. Rolaids) or calcium carbonate (e.g. Tums) can help to minimize cramps during an adventure race and can have an added benefit of reducing GI upset. It is important to note that too much magnesium can lead to diarrhea and too much calcium can lead to constipation. As with any suggestion, it is important to "listen to your body" and see what works best for an individual through trial and error during training and less important races.

Sodium has received a lot of attention recently due to some reports of hyponatremia during marathons. Most studies have found that the incidence of hyponatremia (Na < 135 mmol$\cdot$L^{-1}) is < 5 % in adventure racing and ultra-endurance sports. In general, the risk of hyponatremia increases in those who gain weight during a race, who are less fit, and when hypotonic fluids are readily available (the latter 2 are usually not an issue in ultra-endurance sports). The propensity for hyponatremia is a function of sodium intake and output. The excessive consumption of low sodium beverages (water, soda pop) and those who are high sodium sweaters (white crust on clothes, stinging eyes) are more prone to developing hyponatremia and may require added sodium (tablets, capsules, foods (chips/pretzels)) to prevent hyponatremia during prolonged exercise. On the contrary, it is possible to take too much sodium and become hypernatremic. The latter is more uncommon than hyponatremia, but an excessive weight loss is one risk factor.

> It is impossible to carry even the minimal requirements for a 24 h race on the person and it is essential that support stations are carefully planned or necessary measures are taken to ensure enough fluid intake for the maximal amount of time between a check-point. Filtering or another water purification method may be required.

Hydration is a critical factor in any endurance sport. The recommendations put forth for the triathlete in Chapter 25 are relevant to the ultra-endurance athlete. In addition, there are several unique issues to consider. Firstly, it is impossible to carry even the minimal requirements for a 24 h race on the person (24 kg) and it is essential that support stations are carefully planned and enough fluid is taken for the maximal amount of time between a check-point. There have been many examples where a navigation error has turned a 4 h trek into a 16 h nightmare.

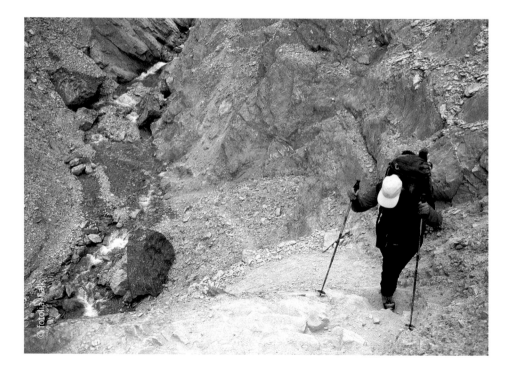

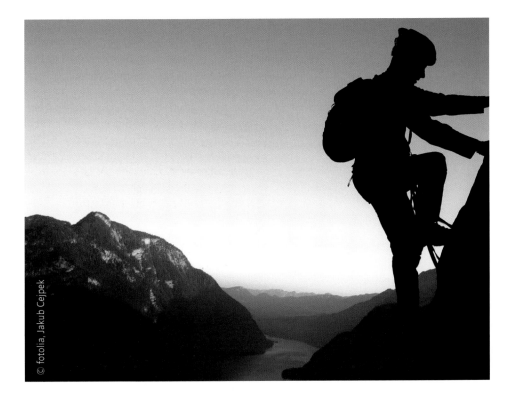

© Fotolia, Jakub Cejpek

In the absence of a suitable alternative filtering or purification method are required. It is critical to choose the filter to match the intended pathogens in the area (e.g. filters work well for larger organisms such as Giardia but are useless for viruses). It is also important to note that iodine is not appropriate for large volume or prolonged consumption of fluid and the water is highly unpalatable. Other practical issues regarding fluid intake include: insulating the drink hose in winter races to prevent freezing, setting up a drink system compatible with paddling (no hands), and changing flavors to prevent taste fatigue. It is also vitally important to bring a variety of foods with varying levels of protein, carbohydrate and fat. Animal studies have shown that consuming very high levels of carbohydrate leads to a subsequent preference for foods higher in fat and protein, and vice versa. One need only try to complete a multi-day stage race on gels, sport drink, and other high carbohydrate foods to experience this phenomenon in reality. Along these lines, human taste is highly individual and it is important to allow for some flexibility to suit the individual tastes of team members in an adventure race. Finally, it is important to consider the palatability and sterility of food when packing for a long trek. For example, pizza in aluminum foil for 8 h in a pack is less than appealing and has the potential for high bacteria counts. Likewise, food not in water-proof bags on the bottom of a kayak or canoe or chocolate bars that melt after a few hours are also not edible. Bars of any sort harden to the consistency of shoe leather in cold races and should be pre-cut into small pieces that can be warmed in the mouth.

In general, it is impossible to provide strict rules for adventure racing and ultra-endurance events; however, following the above guidelines, speaking with experts, and learning what works within the context of one's own body are the keys to successful nutrition. It is likely that the specific person to person nutritional strategies will vary more between any two adventure racers than between any other two athletes in any other sport.

Table 3: Practical tips to maximize fluid and nutrient intake

Challenge to fluid/nutrient consumption	Suggested solution(s)
Nausea	• Practice eating/drinking while training. • Try calcium carbonate, calcium/magnesium, bismuth subsalicylate, or H2 receptor blockers. • Consume small amounts/volumes frequently.
Eating/drinking on the go	• Tape gels to handlebar stem • Use bladder/tube system and bottles accessible on the pack shoulder straps. • Use both water bottles and handlebar mounted fluid systems on the bike. • Have a mixture of 50 – 100 g of food in Velcro pockets on waist belt and pack straps. • Keep food on top of pack or side pockets and practice having others remove it during running.
Winter racing	• Insulate drinking tubes. • Start with warm/hot fluid (longer to freeze). • Break bars into bite size pieces and put into Ziplocs bags • Pack fluids in the middle of clothes for insulation. • Use dry chemical heaters to keep fluid warm. • Keep an emergency non-breakable Thermos of hot fluid (coffee, tea, Ribena, and the like). • Remember that fluid loss can still be high.
Water/food sterility	• Sterilize water bottles and bladders before each use to prevent bacteria build-up. • In longer races know the water pathogens and use the proper filtration or sterilization method. • Do not drink untreated water in most third world countries. • Bring some pre-packaged food to foreign countries. • Use a flip-top protector on the bike water-bottle. • Make sure that food is in water-proof containers on the paddle.
Getting tired of food during the race	• Mix up protein/fat/carbohydrate foods. • Have both savory and sweet foods in your pack and at the transition. • Try to have hot foods at transitions. • Cleanse the palate with carbonated soda. • Brush your teeth.

Chapter 27

Team sports

Stuart Phillips

Classical exercise physiology teaches us that long distance runners and cyclists need to worry about glycogen, that middle distance runners need to worry about lactate, and that sprinters need to be concerned about phosphocreatine. However, what happens when you sprint repeatedly in the context of something such as a soccer match or in a game of ice hockey or basketball? While we have made big strides in understanding the physiology, and thus the nutritional requirements, of team sports we are still hampered in many regards. For example, some fitness components of field-based team sports are poorly understood. In particular, repeated-sprint ability (RSA) is one

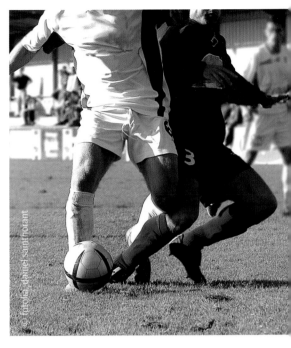

area that has received relatively little research attention. Historically, it has been difficult to investigate the nature of RSA, because of the unpredictability of player movements performed during field-based team sports. However, with improvements in technology, time-motion analysis has allowed researchers to document the detailed movement patterns of team-sport athletes. Studies that have published time-motion analysis during competition, in general, have reported the mean distance and duration of sprints during field-based team sports to be between 10-20 m and 2-3 seconds, respectively. While these sprints are not particularly long, when performed repeatedly they change the pattern of fuel use drastically. In fact, with repeated sprinting one turns into an 'endurance athlete' whose concern for fuel is the same as that of the long distance runner; get more carbohydrate! The figures below show:

- The cellular energy system that fuels a maximal sprint on the 1st, the 3rd, and the nth sprint of sport. Thus, with repeated sprinting you switch from phosphocreatine to aerobic carbohydrate metabolism – i.e., glucose that is burned through oxidative metabolism the same way a long distance runner burns fuel!

- The inset figure shows the fuel we rely on during high intensity work - carbohydrate. In fact, when you're in the 'critical performance zone' (CPZ) and have to sprint all out at any stage of the game, to make a play, then carbohydrate is going to be acutely important.

> As with long-term endurance events, RSA is going to be supported by maximizing carbohydrate intake prior to, during, and after the event to restore and recover.

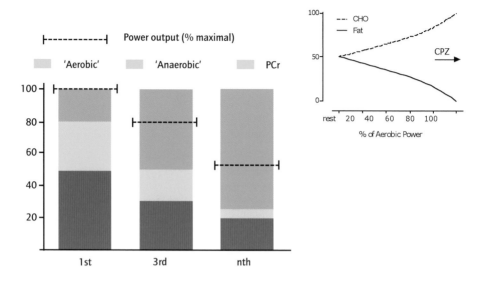

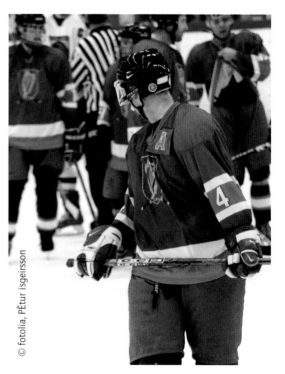

Figure 1. Main: The muscular fuel system that supplies our energy during the 1st, 3rd, and nth sprint during a match. Also, the mean power as a percent of maximal is indicated for each sprint (dashed line). Inset: Balance of fuel utilization in exercise of varying intensity. CPZ – 'critical performance zone'

Time-motion analyses of sports such as soccer, rugby, ice hockey, and basketball show that athletes can cover as much as 12km (soccer), 10km (rugby), 4km (ice hockey), or 2km (basketball). In these sports, the most up-to-date estimates are that one can spend up to 30% (soccer), 25% (rugby), 50% (ice hockey), and 20% (basketball) of your time in what is referred to in the inset of Figure 1 as the CPZ (i.e., a zone in which exercise intensity or movement is most definitely >80% of maximal). It needs to be stressed that even the most intricate time-motion analysis will underestimate the energy requirements of a given sport. For example, running while dribbling results in expenditure of considerably more energy than simply running the same speed without the ball!

© fotolia, PÈtur isgeirsson

Nutritional challenges to RSA in team sports

The biggest nutritional challenges to team sport athletes are not dissimilar to endurance runners or cyclists and would include: getting adequate carbohydrate intake during training to allow maximal performance to enhance training adaptations, getting adequate carbohydrate during a match to maintain glycemia and provide fuel, consumption of adequate carbohydrate and protein in recovery (from matches and strenuous training) to promote muscle glycogen restoration as well as repair/rebalance protein needs which may be elevated. It is also essential to address fluid intake throughout training, competition, and in recovery situations to maximize adaptation, prevent declines in performance, and restore lost fluid, respectively (see Table 1).

> At critical times in team sports, exercise intensities come close to, or even periodically exceed, power outputs of 100% of maximal; at these intensities the fuel used is carbohydrate.

Table 1: Nutritional challenges and solution for RSA in team sports a match

Challenges	Solutions
Fueling during the game	• Try to ingest as close as possible to 40-60 g of carbohydrate/hour but bearing in mind that this may not be possible with intense exercise and with running. • Use drinks, gels, food, whatever your preference. Try out your strategy during a training session to figure out what works best.
Dehydration: Nothing will affect performance faster!	• Assume sweat losses are at least 800ml·h, or 1.5-2.5 times greater in hot environments. • Drink according to environmental conditions – hotter more humid conditions = greater volume. • Aim to achieve fluid balance – i.e., no net weight loss during a match (test during practice).
Avoid muscle cramps during the game	• Causes unknown, but likely related to ionic imbalances: consume drinks containing sodium (20mmol)
Consuming enough carbohydrate during periods of hard training	• Ensure a high carbohydrate diet, which increases with increasing training load: aim for intakes of 6-8 g CHO·kg·d
Consuming adequate protein to promote recovery	• Consumption of a meal containing 25g of high quality protein (milk, eggs, low fat meat) within 1h of completing a training session or a match

A number of field-based studies in soccer players, ice hockey players, basketball players as well as in football players undertaking simulated practices have shown that higher pre-game (i.e., in the 2-3d prior to a game) carbohydrate intakes facilitate improved sport and sport-specific performance.

Table 2: Eating for team sports

Timing	What to eat, when to eat, and why?
Pre-game	• To 'top-off' glycogen stores and prevent hunger, eat 3h before match. • What foods? 60% carb (mostly starch and 2-3g fiber), 25% protein, 15% fat. • Breads, soups, small serving (3oz) of lean meat/fish, vegetables and/or salad - If the players like it, keep doing it! • Water or isotonic Sport drink to achieve free-flowing (urination every 20-30min) clear urine.
During	• Isotonic Sport drink during and at breaks, particularly between periods/halftime • Starch/Sugar snack – Arrowroot cookies, fruit
Post-match	• Eat as soon as possible: rehydrate, refuel, recover • Isotonic Sport drink to match loss – weight change pre- to post-match • Milk (especially chocolate milk) – promotes rehydration and delivers protein to speed recovery • Breads, pasts, rice • Apples, Oranges, Bananas – carbohydrates, some fiber, and vitamins/minerals • Cottage cheese, lean meats, eggs • All of the above MUST be matched to an athlete's playing goals, experience and preferences.

Supplements that may aid performance

Phosphocreatine (PCr) is primarily an energy buffer to defend against reductions in ATP content with any transition in energy requirement, including sprinting. As such, creatine supplementation to increase PCr concentration may offer some advantage to RSA; particularly if creatine facilitates recovery of PCr levels (see Figure 1). Simulated field-based and some actual field-based studies of various sports have shown creatine supplementation to be of benefit for RSA and some sport-specific tasks; however, the balance of evidence is that pre-game creatine loading may have a down side for some athletes in sports with some running component. Body weight increases tend be 1-2kg with creatine loading (a protocol that involves 20-30g of creatine·d^{-1} in 3-4 equal doses for 5d followed by a maintenance dose of 2-5g·d^{-1}). This body mass gain can affect running efficiency and gait kinematics which makes it more difficult for some athletes to compensate for these changes.

> Getting ready to compete in team sports involves consistency and figuring out what certain athletes like. In the end, however, it's all about fluids and carbohydrate before, during and after. Post-match should also emphasize some good high quality protein.

Caffeine is an ergogenic aid that has now been removed from most banned substance lists. As a result, is quite in vogue with many athletes, including those involved in RSA in team sports. This is not surprising since there is little evidence contrary to a larger volume of data that suggests that caffeine in doses from 1-5mg·kg^{-1} 30-90 min prior to or even during an event (prior to substantial fatigue onset) enhances performance.

Bicarbonate or citrate ingestion has been practiced for a long time since it is well recognized that the blood as well as intramuscular pH declines with repeated sprinting. Thus, enhancing the blood buffering capacity by ingestion of bicarbonate (300mg·kg^{-1} which appears to be the most effective dose) or citrate (500 mg·kg^{-1}) at least 1-2h pre-match would appear to offer some benefit. A large number of studies with simulated-match studies have shown some benefit, but more sport-specific research is needed here. Also, the risk of gastrointestinal symptoms with both bicarbonate and citrate appears to be substantial. Chronic ingestion of bicarbonate with high intensity training, however, may allow the athlete to train harder and, in doing so, enhance training adaptations.

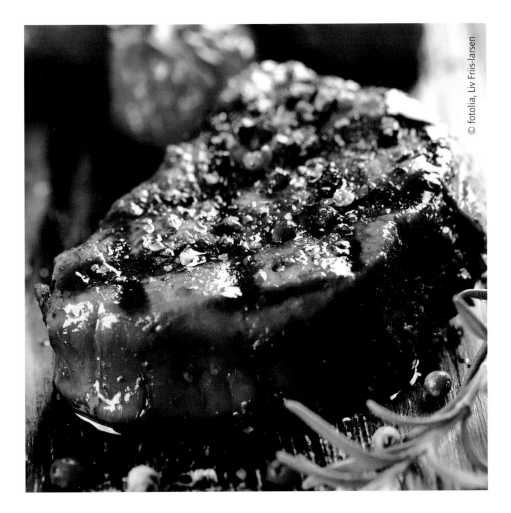

© fotolia, Liv Friis-larsen

Chapter 28

The Future:
Individualizing nutrition & hydration

Dr. Trent Stellingwerff, PhD - Nestlé Research Center, Switzerland

All too often general nutrition advice is followed without particular consideration for how it applies to each individual athlete. One shoe does not fit all. There is more and more of a trend towards individualized advice, and this approach will certainly be the future of sports nutrition. This final chapter will outline some of the practical advice for individualizing and properly fine-tuning and periodizing nutrition (making training specific to the training phase) and hydration recommendations to athletes. This individualized and systematized approach should be undertaken in conjunction with coaches and/or sport scientists (dieticians, nutritionists, and exercise physiologists). This chapter highlights several key nutrition and hydration recommendations outlined in this book and will be further discussed below with practical advice on how to adapt and adjust these to individual athletes.

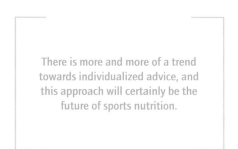

There is more and more of a trend towards individualized advice, and this approach will certainly be the future of sports nutrition.

Implementing and testing new interventions

It is important to experiment with and mimic (practice) any new recommendation (logistics, environment, nutrition, etc.) prior to any major event. Even some of the most scientifically accepted interventions (e.g. glycogen loading prior to an endurance event) may need individual adjustments and piloting to ensure optimal success. Figure 1 below outlines a decision matrix that should be implemented with each new intervention. Although incredibly simple and obvious, in practice it is alarming (even at the elite level) how many athletes and coaches do not fully characterize the individual performance response of a new intervention prior to a major competition. Anticipating all possible outcomes will result in an athlete having full confidence in their unique and individualized approach, which will help them realize their best possible performance for their targeted championship event.

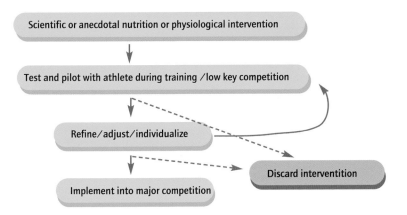

Figure 1. Decision matrix when implementing new interventions

Individualizing and tracking recovery and adaptation

Optimizing recovery via individualized nutritional recommendations and protocols can have a large impact on training load, quality and ultimately performance for a given athlete. All athletes across different sports utilize an incredibly diverse and varied exercise stimulus. Therefore, depending on the previous exercise mode, intensity and duration, the acute recovery nutritional recommendations will also vary. (See Chapters 17-22 for more information on individualized recovery regimes.)

An easy way to track the effectiveness of nutritional and training interventions over time, or identify athletes at-risk for over-reaching or over-training, is through simple questionnaire based approaches. Here are 3 different established and scientifically verified questionnaires that can be utilized:

- **DALDA** - Daily Analysis of Life Demands in Athletes. This 1 page, 34 question analysis can be used daily to track training and life stress in athletes (Rushall 1990).
- **TQR** – Total Quality Recovery. Total quality recovery (TQR) is a concept that looks at daily recovery as a combination of processes and recovery actions and the athlete's perceptions of recovery. It gives coaches and athletes a simple checklist of factors that lead to TQR. Should recovery not be occurring as anticipated, the responsible factor is easily identifiable (Kenntta and Hassmen, 1998).
- **POMS** – Profile of Mood States. Profile Of Mood States (POMS) is a popular tool among sport psychologists who have used it to compare the prevailing moods of non to elite athletes to identify over-reaching and over-training symptoms (Morgan 1980)

Collectively, these approaches and tools can offer a coach/nutritionist a more individualized dimension to their recovery approaches with athletes. At the elite level, nutrition, training and racing interactions need to be highly monitored and continually altered and individualized.

Maximizing aerobic and fat metabolism during endurance training phases

Current carbohydrate (CHO) recommendations contend that endurance athletes should always consume adequate CHO during prolonged exercise training and consume CHO immediately after exercise to ensure subsequent training bouts are conducted in a glycogen-compensated or fed state. However, anecdotal reports from professional cyclists and East African distance runners indicate that some of these athletes purposely and periodically undertake training in either a glycogen-depleted state, or a fasted/water-only state, in an attempt to "force the muscle to adapt to the next level." Recommendations on training with low muscle glycogen are made in Chapter 10.

> Many questions remain on how to optimize aerobic metabolism through training by reducing carbohydrate availability. This is an area of research that will receive a lot of attention in the years to come.

Fasted training is another possible method to induce more aerobic training adaptation, which is physiologically different than low glycogen training. Accordingly, another recent training study examined the effects of fat-metabolism and aerobic muscle markers by having athletes train 3 times per week, for 1 to 2 hours over 6 weeks while either consuming CHO or water (during training) after an overnight fast. Interestingly, after 6 weeks the fasted trained group had an increase in the proteins involved with fat oxidation, but no performance measures were made. Given that this area of research is so young, many questions remain on how to best optimize aerobic and fat oxidation through training without carbohydrate.

The following practical recommendations can currently be made regarding either glycogen and/or fasted training to individualize the approach for each athlete:

- Only apply to and test with athletes who race longer than 30 minutes.
- Periodize fasted or low-glycogen training during general prep phase once or twice every 7 to 10 days.
- For fasted training: Train first thing in the morning. Go straight out the door with just water (or small amount of food)
- For fasted training, gradually increase the length of the training bout, starting with at least 60 minutes, and even incorporate some threshold (not speed) work after several weeks/months. Anecdotally, over time, athletes have been able to do up to 1 hour 45 minutes of running and >3 hours of cycling completely fasted.
- For low-glycogen training, periodize so that speed work is done with high muscle glycogen (to ensure high quality training), and prolonged sub-threshold training is done while in the low-glycogen state (periodically). (See Chapter 10 for more details.)
- Initially practice these nutrition/training techniques over several months prior to lower key races, not right before a major competition.

- These training techniques are another way to provide a "hard" stimulus to your training – but be aware– it is catabolic. This type of training needs to be monitored closely with emphasis on recovery and weight management. (Don't lose too much weight). Though emphasis needs to be on immediate recovery, a bit more recovery time may be needed before next quality session.
- During competition phase, drop all together, or limit to one fasted or low glycogen traininbg session per week.

These recent and emerging scientific findings have caused a degree of uncertainty with regard to the idea that athletes should *always* strive to (endurance) train with ample exogenous (carbohydrate drinks, pre-training meal) and endogenous CHO availability (ample muscle glycogen). Despite the fact that these types of training are both physiologically and psychologically challenging, perhaps athletes may need to periodically cycle glycogen stores and undertake fasted training to maximize the benefits during the endurance training phase. However, whether this nutrition cycling clearly leads to a significant training induced performance benefit compared to standard training regimes remains to be established.

Tracking hydration status and individualizing fluid & fuel intake and pacing targets

Consuming CHO during prolonged endurance exercise can improve performance (see Chapter 4). However, carbohydrate sports drinks fulfill two physiological needs for the endurance athlete: 1) provide fluid and 2) provide energy/fuel. All fueling and hydration scenarios (e.g. predicted race weather conditions) need to be anticipated and practiced by using sports drinks, gels and bars with supplemental water intake to find the athlete's individual tolerance level.

The recent 2007 American College of Sports Medicine position stand.on fluid intake illustrates the need for making fluid intake recommendations according to one's individual sweat rate (Sawka et al 2007). Research has clearly demonstrated that both sweat rates and fluid and fuel intake tolerance are highly individual. There is also an optimal amount of fluid and CHO intake which can improve performance and, conversely, excessive amounts which can cause gastro-intestinal (GI) discomfort and decrease performance. Given that each athlete has his or her own tipping point it would be advantageous to determine the unique and proper balance needed to maximize performance. (see Chapter 21). Therefore, practically speaking, in the 4 to 8 weeks leading into a major endurance competition, athletes should be encouraged to track and record their individual sweat rate and fuel and fluid tolerances during each prolonged training session in, ideally, the anticipated race day weather

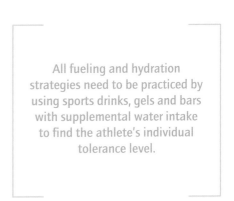

All fueling and hydration strategies need to be practiced by using sports drinks, gels and bars with supplemental water intake to find the athlete's individual tolerance level.

conditions. By measuring pre- and post-training body weight (pounds), and adding fluid intake (quarts), athletes can learn to customize their race day fluid and fueling intakes.

The following is a practical example of estimating the amount of fluid intake per hour needed to prevent a greater than 3% loss in body weight under certain weather conditions. Table 1 (below) outlines several training sessions and race day hydration and sweat rates of an endurance athlete who competed at the 2008 Beijing Olympic Games.

Table 1: Calculated sweat and fluid intake rates during acclimation camp and Beijing Olympic Final

| Parameters | | Singapore Training Camp | | Beijing |
		Workout #1 Aug. 10th	Workout #2 Aug. 12th	Olympic Final Au. 22nd
Weather	Temp (°C)	32°C	28°C	29°C
	Humidity (%)	84 %	86 %	55 %
	Humidex	48	40	36
Pre-weight (kg)		68.1 kg	68.1 kg	67.7 kg
Post-weight (kg)		64.1 kg	66.7kg	65.9 kg
(%BW loss)		(5.9 %)	(2.1%)	(2.6 %)
Weight change		4.0 kg	1.4 kg	1.8 kg
		+	+	+
Total fluids consumed (L)		1.9 L	2.4 L	4.7 L
Total fluid turnover (L or kg)		5.9 L	3.8 L	6.5 L
		/	/	/
Exercise time (h)		3 h	2.25 h	4.1 h
Sweat Rate (ml•h)*		2000ml•h^{-1}	1700ml•h^{-1}	1600ml•h^{-1}
Actual Fluids Intake Rate (ml•h^{-1})		630ml•h^{-1}	1070ml•h^{-1}	1140ml•h^{-1}
Calculated fluid intake rate to prevent >3% BW loss		1270ml•h^{-1}	760ml•h^{-1}	1020ml•h^{-1}

* Urine losses not accounted for in sweat rate; 1 L water = 1 kg; BW - body weight; Temp - Temperature

An individualized hydration and fueling plan was developed for this athlete by repeatedly collecting data on the sweat rate and fluid and carbohydrate intake rates in the 4 to 6 weeks leading up to the Olympic Games, and by incorporating the qualitative feedback on GI tolerance to the fluid and carbohydrate intake. This plan was successfully implemented in very difficult environmental conditions on competition day.

Gastro-intestinal tract adaptation

Numerous anecdotal reports support the idea that an individual's GI tract can be trained and adapted to handle the intake of large amounts of CHO and fluid during exercise – providing more rationale for the need to documenting and evaluating different nutritional interventions between training and racing situations. (See Chapter 21 for more information.) Accordingly, recent published data has suggested that the GI tolerance to large amounts of CHO intake can be optimized and adapted, although the ultimate amount appears to be very individual (Jeukendrup 2004). Therefore, during the preceding competitions and in the immediate 2 to 4 weeks prior to a major competition, athletes should be encouraged to consistently consume fluids and CHO during all prolonged training sessions to become very accustomed to and comfortable with the CHO-based sports drinks that will be used on competition day. Recent data has shown that not only can fluid tolerance improve through repeated practice, but the intestinal CHO transporters can also be

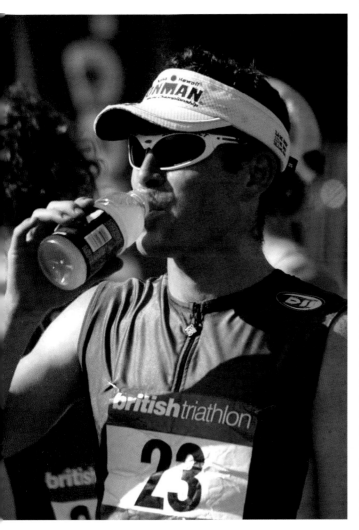

up-regulated and increased through several weeks of CHO intake, albeit in a rodent model. Given that most of the limited and existing mechanistic data on gut adaptation and up-regulation of CHO intestinal transporters is from rodent studies, this area of gut adaptation for endurance athletes appears ripe for further scientific examination.

When to seek expert advice

In general, as long as individuals adhere to a healthy and well-balanced diet with attention to nutritional recovery, and obtain ideal rest and recovery from training, then highly specialized nutritional advice is normally not warranted. Nearly all of the dietary recommendations that most athletes need can be found within this book. However, for many elite athletes and a small percentage of the others, there are unique and specific situations that will need to be properly addressed by qualified and experienced sports nutrition professionals. The list below highlights some of the situations for which an expert opinion may be needed:

- Are you consistently very fatigued every single day during a hard training phase?
- Do you continually get run-down and sick? (decreased immune function?)
- Do you tend to run out of fuel in workouts or afternoon runs, and feel lightheaded or like you have no energy?
- Do you have wild fluctuations in body weight throughout the training year (greater than a 5% gain or loss in body weight)?
- Do you have a very hard time trying to maintain a lean and competitive physique in a healthy manner?
- Have you had problems with iron-deficiency (anemia) on several occasions?
- (For female athletes) Have you experienced amenorrhea (no menstrual cycle) for longer than a continuous 3 or 4 month length of time?
- After a hard work-out or race, do you have severe muscle soreness for several days on end?

Summary

For elite athletes, a comprehensive, long-term approach to nutrition and training interactions need to be carefully planned and monitored between the coach, athlete and nutrition expert. The concept of periodizing nutrition throughout the varied training year is scientifically under-addressed (Stellingwerff et al 2006). Future developments should seek to integrate practical nutrition and training recommendations into a periodized and individualized approach for each athlete. Emerging nutrition and training methods, such as low-glycogen or fasted training, do not negate the importance of good overall nutrition for training. Instead, they place more emphasis on the intelligent periodization of training and nutrition interactions, which are specific to the training session and the desired physiological adaptation. Test and mimic all planned interventions prior to competition. Anticipating all possible outcomes will result in athletes having full confidence in their unique and individualized approach, which will help them realize their best possible performance for their targeted championship event.

References

Chapter 1

Dill, Edwards & Talbott (1932). Factors limiting the capacity for work. *J Physiol*, 49-62.

Larrabee (1902). Leucocytosis after violent exercise. *J Med Research, 7*, 76–82.

Levine, Gordon & Derick (1924). Some changes in chemical constituents of blood following a marathon race. *JAMA, 82*, 1778-1779.

Mottram (1988). *Drugs in sport*. Champaign, IL: Human Kinetics.

Carpenter (1931). The fuel of muscular activity in man. *J Nutr, 4*, 281-304.

Terlung & Horton (Eds.). (1988). Exercise, Nutrition and Energy Metabolism. New York: MacMillan.

Chapter 2

Burke, Cox, Cummings & Desbrow (2001). Guidelines for daily carbohydrate intake: do athletes achieve them? *Sports Med, 31*, 267-299

Burke, Slater, Broad, Haulka, Modulon & Hopkins (2003). Eating patterns and meal frequency of elite Australian athletes. *Int. J. Sports Nutr. Exerc. Metab, 13*, 1-19.

Saris, Van Erp-Baart, Brouns, Westerterp & Ten Hoor (1989). Study on food intake and energy expenditure during extreme sustained exercise: the Tour de France. *Int. J. Sports Med, 10,* 26-31.

Chapter 3

Achten & Jeukendrup (2003). Effects of pre-exercise ingestion of carbohydrate on glycaemic and insulinaemic responses during subsequent exercise at differing intensities. *Eur J Appl Physiol, 88*(4-5), 466-471.

Balsom, Wood, Olsson & Ekblom (1999). Carbohydrate intake and multiple sprint sports: with special reference to football (soccer). *Int J Sports Med, 20*(1), 48-52.

Bangsbo, Nørregaard & Thorsøe (1992). The effect of carbohydrate diet on intermittent exercise performance. *Int J Sports Med, 13*(2), 152-157.

Casey, Mann, Banister, Fox, Morris, Macdonald, et al. (2000). Effect of carbohydrate ingestion on glycogen resynthesis in human liver and skeletal muscle, measured by (13)C MRS. *Am J Physiol Endocrinol Metab, 278*(1), E65-75.

Chryssanthopoulos, Hennessy & Williams (1994). The influence of pre-exercise glucose ingestion on endurance running capacity. *Br J Sports Med, 28*(2), 105-109.

Fallowfield, Williams & Singh (1995). The influence of ingesting a carbohydrate-electrolyte beverage during 4 hours of recovery on subsequent endurance capacity. *Int J Sport Nutr, 5*(4), 285-299.

Jentjens, Cale, Gutch & Jeukendrup (2003). The effects of different amounts of pre-exercise carbohydrate feeding on metabolism and cycling performance. *Eur J Appl Physiol. 88:* 444-52.

Jentjens & Jeukendrup (2002b). Prevalence of hypoglycemia following pre-exercise carbohydrate ingestion is not accompanied by higher insulin sensitivity. *Int J Sport Nutr Exerc Metab, 12*(4), 398-413.

Jentjens & Jeukendrup (2003). Effects of pre-exercise ingestion of trehalose, galactose and glucose on subsequent metabolism and cycling performance. *Eur J Appl Physiol, 88*(4-5), 459-465.

Montain, Hopper, Coggan & Coyle (1991). Exercise metabolism at different time intervals after a meal. *J Appl Physiol, 70*(2), 882-888.

Moseley, Lancaster & Jeukendrup (2003). Effects of timing of pre-exercise ingestion of carbohydrate on subsequent metabolism and cycling performance. *Eur J Appl Physiol, 88*(4-5), 453-458.

Nicholas, Green, Hawkins & Williams (1997). Carbohydrate intake and recovery of intermittent running capacity. *Int J Sport Nutr, 7*, 251-260.

Wee, Williams, Gray & Horabin (1999). Influence of high and low glycemic index meals on endurance running capacity. *Med Sci Sports Exerc, 31*(3), 393-399.

Wright, Sherman & Dernbach (1991). Carbohydrate feedings before, during, or in combinatio improve cycling endurance performance. *J Appl Physiol, 71*(3), 1082-1088.

Chapter 4

Carter, Jeukendrup, Mundel & Jones (2003). Carbohydrate supplementation improves moderate and high-intensity exercise in the heat. *Pflugers Arch, 446*(2), 211-219.

Currell, Conway & Jeukendrup (2009). Carbohydrate ingestion improves performance of a new reliable test of soccer performance. *Int J Sport Nutr Exerc Metab, 19*(1), 34-46.

Currell & Jeukendrup (2008). Superior endurance performance with ingestion of multiple transportable carbohydrates. *Med Sci Sports Exerc, 40*(2), 275-281.

Jeukendrup & Jentjens (2000). Oxidation of carbohydrate feedings during prolonged exercise: current thoughts, guidelines and directions for future research. *Sports Med, 29*, 407-424.

Jeukendrup (2004). Carbohydrate intake during exercise and performance. *Nutrition, 20*(7-8), 669-677.

Jeukendrup, Jentjens & Moseley (2005). Nutritional considerations in triathlon. *Sports Med, 35*(2), 163-181.

Chapter 5

Currell & Jeukendrup (2008). Superior endurance performance with ingestion of multiple transportable carbohydrates. *Med Sci Sports Exerc, 40*(2), 275-281.

Jeukendrup & Moseley (Epub DOI: 10.1111/j.1600-0838.2008.00862.x). Multiple transportable carbohydrates enhance gastric emptying and fluid delivery. *Scand J Med Sci Sports.*

Jeukendrup, Moseley, Mainwaring, Samuels, Perry & Mann (2006). Exogenous carbohydrate oxidation during ultraendurance exercise. *J Appl Physiol, 100*(4), 1134-1141.

Noakes (2007a). Drinking guidelines for exercise: what evidence is there that athletes should drink "as much as tolerable", "to replace the weight lost during exercise" or "ad libitum"? *J Sports Sci, 25*(7), 781-796.

Noakes (2007b). Hydration in the marathon: using thirst to gauge safe fluid replacement. *Sports Med, 37*(4-5), 463-466.

Sawka, Burke, Eichner, Maughan, Montain & Stachenfeld (2007a). American College of Sports Medicine position stand. Exercise and fluid replacement. *Med Sci Sports Exerc, 39*(2), 377-390.

Sawka & Noakes (2007b). Does dehydration impair exercise performance? *Med Sci Sports Exerc, 39*(8), 1209-1217.

Chapter 6

Achten & Jeukendrup (2003a). The effect of pre-exercise carbohydrate feedings on the intensity that elicits maximal fat oxidation. *J Sports Sci, 21*(12), 1017-1024.

Achten & Jeukendrup (2003b). Maximal fat oxidation during exercise in trained men. *Int J Sports Med, 24*(8), 603-608.

Achten, Venables & Jeukendrup (2003c). Fat oxidation rates are higher during running compared with cycling over a wide range of intensities. *Metabolism, 52*(6), 747-752.

Astrup (1993). Dietary composition, substrate balances and body fat in subjects with a predisposition to obesity. *Int J Obes Relat Metab Disord, 17* Suppl 3, 32-36; discussion 41-32.

De Bock, Derave, Eijnde, Hesselink, Koninckx, Rose, et al. (2008). Effect of training in the fasted state on metabolic responses during exercise with carbohydrate intake. *J Appl Physiol, 104*(4), 1045-1055.

Holloszy & Coyle (1984). Adaptations of skeletal muscle to endurance exercise and their metabolic consequences. *J Appl Physiol, 56*(4), 831-838.

Jeukendrup & Aldred (2004). Fat supplementation, health, and endurance performance. *Nutrition, 20*(7-8), 678-688.

Jeukendrup & Wallis (2005). Measurement of substrate oxidation during exercise by means of gas exchange measurements. *Int J Sports Med, 26* Suppl 1, 28-37.

Venables, Achten & Jeukendrup (2005). Determinants of fat oxidation during exercise in healthy men and women: a cross-sectional study. *J Appl Physiol, 98*(1), 160-167.

Venables, Hulston, Cox & Jeukendrup (2008). Green tea extract ingestion, fat oxidation, and glucose tolerance in healthy humans. *Am J Clin Nutr, 87*(3), 778-784.

Chapter 7

Burke (2007). *Practical Sports Nutrition*. Champaign, IL: Human Kinetics.

Burke, Kiens, Ivy (2004). Carbohydrates and fat for training and recovery. *J Sports Sci, 22*(1), 15-30.

Shirreffs, Armstrong, Cheuvront (2004). Fluid and electrolyte needs for preparation and recovery from training and competition. *J Sports Sci, 22*(1), 57-63.

Chapter 8

Afaghi, O'Connor, et al. (2007). High-glycemic-index carbohydrate meals shorten sleep onset. *Am J Clin Nutr, 85*(2), 426-430.

Arnulf, Quintin, et al. (2002). Mid-morning tryptophan depletion delays REM sleep onset in healthy subjects. *Neuropsychopharmacology, 27*(5), 843-851.

Atkinson, Drust, et al. (2003). The relevance of melatonin to sports medicine and science. *Sports Med, 33*(11), 809-831.

Bent, Padula, et al. (2006). Valerian for sleep: a systematic review and meta-analysis. *Am J Med, 119*(12), 1005-1012.

Hartmann (1982). Effects of L-tryptophan on sleepiness and on sleep. *J Psychiatr Res, 17*(2), 107-113.

Horne & Shackell (1987). Slow wave sleep elevations after body heating: proximity to sleep and effects of aspirin. *Sleep, 10*(4), 383-392.

Postolache & Oren (2005). Circadian phase shifting, alerting, and antidepressant effects of bright light treatment. *Clin Sports Med, 24*(2), 381-413, xii.

Reilly & Deykin (1983). Effects of partial sleep loss on subjective states, psychomotor and physical performance tests. *Journal of Human Movement Studies, 9*, 157-170.

Reilly & Edwards (2007). Altered sleep-wake cycles and physical performance in athletes. *Physiol Behav, 90*(2-3), 274-284.

Roky, Chapotot, et al. (2001). Sleep during Ramadan intermittent fasting. *J Sleep Res, 10*(4), 319-327.

Rundell, Lester, et al. (1972). Alcohol and sleep in young adults. *Psychopharmacologia, 26*(3), 201-218.

Sinnerton & Reilly (1992). Effects of sleep loss and time of day in swimmers. In D. Maclaren, T. Reilly & A. Lees (Eds.), *Biomechanics and medicine in swimming: Swimming Science IV* (pp. 399-405). London: Routledge.

Sung & Tochihara (2000). Effects of bathing and hot footbath on sleep in winter. *J Physiol Anthropol Appl Human Sci, 19*(1), 21-27.

Chapter 9

Hartman, Tang, Wilkinson, Tarnopolsky, Lawrence, Fullerton, et al. (2007). Consumption of fat-free fluid milk after resistance exercise promotes greater lean mass accretion than does consumption of soy or carbohydrate in young, novice, male weightlifters. *Am J Clin Nutr, 86*(2), 373-381.

Kreider (1999). Dietary supplements and the promotion of muscle growth with resistance exercise. *Sports Med, 27*(2), 97-110.

Phillips (2006). Dietary protein for athletes: from requirements to metabolic advantage. *Appl Physiol Nutr Metab, 31*(6), 647-654.

Phillips (2004). Protein requirements and supplementation in strength sports. *Nutrition, 20*(7-8), 689-695.

Rowlands & Thomson (2009). Effects of beta-hydroxy-beta-methylbutyrate supplementation during resistance training on strength, body composition, and muscle damage in trained and untrained young men: a meta-analysis. *J Strength Cond Res, 23*(3), 836-846.

Tang, Moore, Kujbida, Tarnopolsky & Phillips (2009). Ingestion of whey hydrolysate, casein, or soy protein isolate: effects on mixed muscle protein synthesis at rest and following resistance exercise in young men. *J Appl Physiol, 107*(3), 987-992.

Tang & Phillips (2009). Maximizing muscle protein anabolism: the role of protein quality. *Curr Opin Clin Nutr Metab Care, 12*(1), 66-71.

Tarnopolsky (2004). Protein requirements for endurance athletes. *Nutrition, 20*(7-8), 662-668.

Tarnopolsky, Parise, Yardley, Ballantyne, Olatinji & Phillips (2001). Creatine-dextrose and protein-dextrose induce similar strength gains during training. *Med Sci Sports Exerc, 33*(12), 2044-2052.

Tarnopolsky, Bosman, Macdonald, Vandeputte, Martin, Roy (1997). Postexercise protein-carbohydrate and carbohydrate supplements increase muscle glycogen in men and women. *J Appl Physiol, 83*(6), 1877-1883.

Wilkinson, Tarnopolsky, Macdonald, Macdonald, Armstrong, Phillips (2007). Consumption of fluid skim milk promotes greater muscle protein accretion after resistance exercise than does consumption of an isonitrogenous and isoenergetic soy-protein beverage. *Am J Clin Nutr, 85*(4), 1031-1040.

Chapter 10

Bergstrom, Hermansen, Hultman & Saltin (1967). Diet, muscle glycogen and physical performance. *Acta Physiol Scand, 71*, 140-150.

Bergstrom & Hultman (1966). The effect of exercise on muscle glycogen and electrolytes in normals. *Scand J Clin Lab Invest, 18*, 16-20

Bergstrom & Hultman (1967a). A study of the glycogen metabolism during exercise in man. *Scand J Clin Lab Invest, 19*, 218-228.

Bergstrom & Hultman (1967b). Synthesis of muscle glycogen in man after glucose and fructose infusion. *Acta Med Scand, 182*, 93-107.

Bernard (1858). Nouvelles recherches expérimentales sur les phénomènes glycogeniques du foie. *Comptes rendus de la Société de biologie, 2*, 1-7.

Blomstrand & Saltin (1999). Effect of muscle glycogen on glucose, lactate and amino acid metabolism during exercise and recovery in human subjects. *J Physiol, 514* (Pt 1), 293-302.

Hansen, Fischer, Plomgaard, Andersen, Saltin & Pedersen (2005). Skeletal muscle adaptation: training twice every second day vs. training once daily. *J Appl Physiol, 98*, 93-99

Hultman & Bergstrom (1967). Muscle glycogen synthesis in relation to diet studied in normal subjects. *Acta Med Scand, 182*, 109-117.

Narkar, Downes, Yu, Embler, Wang, Banayo, et al. (2008). AMPK and PPARdelta agonists are exercise mimetics. *Cell, 134*, 405-415.

Steensberg, Van Hall, Keller, Osada, Schjerling, Pedersen, et al. (2002). Muscle glycogen content and glucose uptake during exercise in humans: influence of prior exercise and dietary manipulation. *J Physiol, 541*, 273-281.

Young (1957). Claude Bernard and the discovery of glycogen; a century of retrospect. *Br Med J, 1*, 1431-1437.

Chapter 11

Tipton & Witard (2007). Protein requirements and recommendations for athletes: Relevance of ivory tower arguments for practical recommendations. *Clinics in Sports Medicine, 26*(1), 17-36

Hawley, Tipton & Millard-Stafford (2006). Promoting training adaptations through nutritional interventions. *J. Sports Sci, 24*, 709-721

Tipton & Sharp (2005). The response of intracellular signaling and muscle protein metabolism to nutrition and exercise. *Eur. J. Sports Sci, 5*, 107-121.

Tipton & Wolfe (2004). Protein and amino acids for athletes. *J. Sports Sci, 22*(1), 65-79.

Chapter 12

Currell & Jeukendrup (2008). Superior endurance performance with ingestion of multiple transportable carbohydrates. *Med Sci Sports Exerc, 40*, 275-281.

Jentjens & Jeukendrup (2005). High rates of exogenous carbohydrate oxidation from a mixture of glucose and fructose ingested during prolonged cycling exercise. *Br J Nutr, 93*, 485-492.

Jeukendrup (2008). Carbohydrate feeding during exercise. *European Journal of Sport Science, 8*, 77-86.

Jeukendrup & Moseley (Epub DOI: 10.1111/j.1600-0838.2008.00862.x). Multiple transportable carbohydrates enhance gastric emptying and fluid delivery. *Scand J Med Sci Sports.*

Rowlands, Wallis, Shaw, Jentjens & Jeukendrup (2005). Glucose polymer molecular weight does not affect exogenous carbohydrate oxidation. *Med Sci Sports Exerc, 37*, 1510-1516.

Chapter 13

American College of Sports Medicine (ACSM) (2007). Position stand: exercise and fluid replacement. *Med Sci Sports Exerc, 39*, 377-390.

Braun, Koehler, Geyer, Kleinert, Mester & Schaenzer (2009). Dietary Supplement Use Among Elite Young German Athletes. *Int J Sp Nutr Exerc Met, 19*, 97-109.

Braun, Koehler, Geyer, Thevis & Schaenzer (publication in progress). Dietary supplement use of Olympic German athletes.

Burke, Millet & Tarnopolsky (2007). Nutrition for distance events. *J Sp Sci, 25*, 29-38.

European Comission (2001). *Report of the Scientific Committee on Food on composition and specification of food intended to meet the expenditure of intense muscular effort, especially for sportsmen.* Retrieved March 10, 2009, from
http://ec.europa.eu/food/fs/sc/scf/out64_en.pdf

European Food Safety Authority, Scientific Panel on Dietetic products, nutrition and allergies (NDA) and Scientific Committee on Food (SCF) (2006). *Tolerable upper intake levels for vitamins and minerals.* Retrieved March 10, 2009, from
http://www.efsa.europa.eu/EFSA/efsa_locale-1178620753812_1178633962601.htm

Geyer, Parr, Koehler, Mareck, Schaenzer & Thevis (2008). Nutritional supplements cross-contaminated and faked with doping substance. *J Mass Spectrom, 43*, 892–902.

Hawley, Gibala & Bermon (2007). Innovations in athletic preparation: Role of substrate availability to modify training adaptation and performance. *J Sp Sci, 25*, 115-124.

Jeukendrup (2008). Carbohydrate feeding during exercise. *European Journal of Sport Science, 8,* 77-86.

Maughan, Depiesse & Geyer (2007). The use of dietary supplements by athletes. *J Sp Sci, 25,* 103-13.

Tarnopolsky (2008). Building Muscle: nutrition to maximize bulk and strength adaptations to resistance exercise training. *European Journal of Sport Science, 8,* 67-76.

Tipton (2008). Protein for adaptations to exercise training. *European Journal of Sport Science, 8,* 107-118.

Chapter 14

Geyer, Bredehoft, Marek, Parr & Schanzer (2002). Hohe Dosen des Anabolikums Metandienon in Nahrungsergänzungsmitteln. *Deutsche Apotheker Zeitung, 142, 29*

Geyer, Parr, Mareck, Reinhart, Schrader & Schänzer (2004). Analysis of non-hormonal nutritional supplements for anabolic-androgenic steroids - results of an international study. *Int J Sports Med, 25,*124-9.

Harris R. C., Almada, Harris D. B., Dunnett & Hespel (2004). The creatine content of Creatine SerumTM and the change in the plasma concentration with ingestion of a single dose. *J Sports Sci, 22,* 851–857

Huang, Johnson & Pipe (2006). The use of dietary supplements and medications by Canadian athletes at the Atlanta and Sydney Olympic Games. *Clin J Sports Med, 16,* 27-33.

Krishnan, Feng & Gordon (2009). Prolonged intrahepatic cholestasis and renal failure secondary to anabolic androgenic steroid-enriched dietary supplements. *J Clin Gastroenterol, 43,* 672-675.

Maughan (2005). Contamination of dietary supplements and positive drugs tests in sport. *J Sports Sci, 23,* 883-889.

Maughan, Depiesse & Geyer (2007). The use of dietary supplements by athletes. *J Sports Sci, 25,* 103-113.

Watson, Judkins, Houghton, Russell & Maughan (2009). Supplement contamination: detection of nandrolone metabolites in urine after administration of small doses of a nandrolone precursor. *Med Sci Sports Exerc, 41,* 766-772.

Chapter 15

Gleeson (Ed.). (2005). *Immune Function in Sport and Exercise.* Edinburgh: Elsevier.

Nieman & Pedersen (Eds.). (2000). *Nutrition and Exercise Immunology.* Boca Raton: CRC Press.

Calder, Field & Gill (2002). *Nutrition and Immune Function.* Oxford: CABI Publishing.

Gleeson, Nieman & Pedersen (2004). Exercise, nutrition and immune function. *Journal of Sports Sciences, 22*(1), 115-125.

Umeda, Nakaji, Shimoyama, Kojima, Yamamoto & Sugawara (2004). Adverse effects of energy restriction on changes in immunoglobulins and complements during weight reduction in judoists. *Journal of Sports Medicine and Physical Fitness, 44*(3), 328-334.

Yaegaki, Umeda, Takahashi, Matsuzaka, Sugawara, Shimaya, et al. (2007). Change in the capability of reactive oxygen species production by neutrophils following weight reduction in female judoists. *British Journal of Sports Medicine, 41*(5), 322-327.

Halson, Lancaster, Achten, Gleeson & Jeukendrup (2004). Effect of carbohydrate supplementation on performance and carbohydrate oxidation following intensified cycling training. *Journal of Applied Physiology, 97*, 1245-1253.

Gleeson (2006). Can nutrition limit exercise-induced immunodepression? *Nutrition Reviews, 64*(3), 1-13.

Nieman (2008). Immunonutrition support for athletes. *Nutrition Reviews, 66*(6), 310-320.

Bishop, Blannin, Armstrong, Rickman & Gleeson (2000). Carbohydrate and fluid intake affect the saliva flow rate and IgA response to cycling. *Medicine and Science in Sports and Exercise, 32*(12), 2046-2051.

Fischer, Hiscock, Penkowa, Basu, Vessby, Kallner, et al. (2004). Supplementation with Vitamins C and E inhibits the release of interleukin-6 from contracting human skeletal muscle. *Journal of Physiology, 558*(2), 633-645.

Davison & Gleeson (2006). The effect of 2 weeks vitamin C supplementation on immunoendocrine responses to 2.5 h cycling exercise in man. *European Journal of Applied Physiology, 97*(4), 454-461.

Peters (2000). Vitamins, immunity, and Infection risk in athletes. In Nieman & Pedersen (Eds.), *Nutrition and Exercise Immunology* (pp. 109-136). Boca Raton: CRC Press.

Chapter 16

Nieman (1997). Immune response to heavy exertion. *J Appl Physiol, 82*, 1385-1394.

Nieman (2000). Is infection risk linked to exercise workload? *Med Sci Sports Exerc, 32* (7), 406-411.

Nieman (2008). Immunonutrition support for athletes. *Nutr Rev, 66*(6), 310-320.

Nieman & Bishop (2006). Nutritional strategies to counter stress to the immune system in athletes, with special reference to football. *J Sports Sci, 24*, 763-772.

Gleeson & Thomas (2008). Exercise and immune function. Is there any evidence for probiotic benefit for sports people? *Compl Nutr, 8*(3), 35-37.

Cox, Pyne, Saunders & Fricker (in press). Oral administration of the probiotic Lactobacillus fermentum VRI-003 and mucosal immunity in endurance athletes. *Br J Sports Med.*

Nieman, Henson, Maxwell, Williams, McAnulty, Jin, et al. (2009). Effects of quercetin and EGCG on mitochondrial biogenesis and immunity. *Med Sci Sports Exerc, 41*(7), 1467-75.

Nieman, Henson, McMahon, Wrieden, Davis, Murphy, et al. (2008). Effects of ,-glucan on immune function and upper respiratory tract infections in endurance athletes. *Med Sci Sports Exerc, 40*, 1463-1471.

Nieman, Henson, Gross, Jenkins, Davis, Murphy, et al. (2007). Quercetin reduces illness but not immune perturbations after intensive exercise. *Med Sci Sports Exerc, 39*, 1561-1569.

Chapter 17

Harger-Domitrovich, McClaughry, Gaskill & Ruby (2007). Exogenous carbohydrate spares muscle glycogen in men and women during 10 h of exercise. *Med Sci Sports Exerc, 39*(12), 2171-2179.

M'Kaouar, Péronnet, Massicotte & Lavoie (2004). Gender difference in the metabolic response to prolonged exercise with [13C]glucose ingestion. *Eur J Appl Physiol, 92*(4-5), 462-469.

Riddell, Partington, Stupka, Armstrong, Rennie & Tarnopolsky (2003). Substrate utilization during exercise performed with and without glucose ingestion in female and male endurance trained athletes. *Int J Sport Nutr Exerc Metab, 13*(4), 407-421.

Romijn, Coyle, Sidossis, Gastaldelli, Horowitz, Endert, et al. (1993). Regulation of endogenous fat and carbohydrate metabolism in relation to exercise intensity and duration. *Am J Physiol, 265*(3 Pt 1), 380-391.

Romijn, Coyle, Sidossis, Rosenblatt & Wolfe (2000). Substrate metabolism during different exercise intensities in endurance-trained women. *J Appl Physiol, 88*(5), 1707-1714.

Tarnopolsky, MacDougall, Atkinson, Tarnopolsky & Sutton (1990). Gender differences in substrate for endurance exercise. *J Appl Physiol, 68*(1), 302-308.

Tarnopolsky, Atkinson, Phillips & MacDougall (1995). Carbohydrate loading and metabolism during exercise in men and women. *J Appl Physiol, 78*(4), 1360-1368.

Tarnopolsky, Bosman, Macdonald, Vandeputte, Martin & Roy (1997). Postexercise protein-carbohydrate and carbohydrate supplements increase muscle glycogen in men and women. *J Appl Physiol, 83*(6), 1877-1883.

Tarnopolsky (2008). Sex differences in exercise metabolism and the role of 17-beta estradiol. *Med Sci Sports Exerc, 40*(4), 648-654.

Timmons, Bar-Or & Riddell (2007). Energy substrate utilization during prolonged exercise with and without carbohydrate intake in preadolescent and adolescent girls [Electronic version]. *J Appl Physiol, 103*(3), 995-1000.

Wallis, Dawson, Achten, Webber & Jeukendrup (2006). Metabolic response to carbohydrate ingestion during exercise in males and females [Electronic version]. *Am J Physiol Endocrinol Metab, 290*(4), 708-715.

Chapter 18

Carter, Jeukendrup, Mann & Jones (2004a). The effect of glucose infusion on glucose kinetics during a 1-h time trial. *Med Sci Sports Exerc, 36*, 1543-1550.

Carter, Jeukendrup & Jones (2004b). The effect of carbohydrate mouth rinse on 1-h cycle time trial performance. *Med Sci Sports Exerc, 36*, 2107-2111.

Chambers, Bridge & Jones (2009). Carbohydrate sensing in the human mouth: effects on exercise performance and brain activity. *J Physiol, 587*, 1779-1794.

Jeukendrup, Brouns, Wagenmakers & Saris (1997). Carbohydrate-electrolyte feedings improve 1 h time trial cycling performance. *Int J Sports Med, 18*, 125-129.

Lieberman (2003). Nutrition, brain function and cognitive performance. *Appetite, 40*, 245-54.

Liu, Gao, Liu & Fox (2000). The temporal response of the brain after eating revealed by functional MRI. *Nature, 405*(6790), 1058-1062.

Meeusen & Watson (2007). Amino acids and the brain: Do they play a role in "central fatigue"? *Int J Sports Nutr Exerc Metab, 17* (Suppl), 37-46.

Roelands, Hasegawa, Watson, Piacentini, Buyse, De Schutter, et al. (2008). The effects of acute dopamine reuptake inhibition on performance. *Med Sci Sports Exerc, 40,* 879-885.

Watson, Hasegawa, Roelands, Piacentini, Looverie & Meeusen (2005). Acute dopamine/noradrenaline reuptake inhibition enhances human exercise performance in warm, but not temperate conditions. *J Physiol, 565,* 873-883.

Chapter 19

Stubbs, Harbron, Murgatroyd & Prentice (1995a). Covert manipulation of dietary fat and energy density: effect on substrate flux and food intake in men eating ad libitum. *Am J Clin Nutr, 62,* 316-329.

Stubbs, Ritz, Coward & Prentice (1995b). Covert manipulation of the ratio of dietary fat to carbohydrate and energy density: effect on food intake and energy balance in free-living men eating ad libitum. *Am J Clin Nutr, 62,* 330-337.

Stubbs, Harbron & Prentice (1996). Covert manipulation of the dietary fat to carbohydrate ratio of isoenergetically dense diets: effect on food intake in feeding men ad libitum. *Int J Obes Relat Metab Disord, 20,* 651-660.

Chapter 20

Layman, Evans, Baum, Seyler, Erickson & Boileau (2005). Dietary protein and exercise have additive effects on body composition during weight loss in adult women. *J Nutr, 135,* 1903-1910.

Walberg, Leidy, Sturgill, Hinkle, Ritchey & Sebolt (1988). Macronutrient content of a hypoenergy diet affects nitrogen retention and muscle function in weight lifters. *Int J Sports Med, 9,* 261-266.

Mourier, Bigard, De Kerviler, Roger, Legrand & Guezennec (1997). Combined effects of caloric restriction and branched-chain amino acid supplementation on body composition and exercise performance in elite wrestlers. *Int J Sports Med, 18,* 47-55.

Forbes (2000). Body fat content influences the body composition response to nutrition and exercise. *Ann N Y Acad Sci, 904,* 359-365.

Chapter 21

Pfeiffer, B., Cotterill, A., Grathwohl D., Stellingwerff T. & Jeukendrup A. E. The effect of carbohydrate gels on gastrointestinal tolerance during a 16-km run. (2009) *Int J Sport Nutr Exerc Metab. 19:*485-503.

Brouns & Beckers (1993). Is the gut an athletic organ? Digestion, absorption and exercise. *Sports Med, 15,* 242-257.

Lambert, Lang, Bull, Eckerson, Lanspa & O'Brien (2008). Fluid tolerance while running: Effect of repeated trials. *Int J Sports Med.*

Peters, Van Schelven, Verstappen, De Boer, Bol, Erich, et al. (1993). Gastrointestinal problems as a function of carbohydrate supplements and mode of exercise. *Med Sci Sports Exerc, 25,* 1211-1224.

Chapter 23

Burke, Kiens & Ivy (2004). Carbohydrates and fat for training and recovery. *J Sports Sci, 22,* 15-30.

Jentjens & Jeukendrup (2003). Determinants of post-exercise glycogen synthesis during short-term recovery. *Sports Med, 33,* 117-144.

McNaughton (2000). Bicarbonate and citrate. In R. J. Maughan (Ed.), *Nutrition in Sport* (pp. 393-404). Oxford: Blackwell.

Stellingwerff, Boit & Res (2007). Nutritional strategies to optimize training and racing in middle-distance athletes. *J Sports Sci, 25,* 17-28.

Tarnopolsky (1999). Protein metabolism in strength and endurance activities. In D. R. Lamb, R. Murray, I.N. Carmel (Eds.), *Perspectives in Exercise Science and Sports Medicine: The Metabolic Basis of Performance in Exercise and Sport* (pp. 125-164). Traverse City, MI: Cooper Publishing Group.

Chapter 28

Jeukendrup (2008). Carbohydrate feeding during exercise. *European Journal of Sport Science, 8,* 77-86.

Kenntta & Hassmen (1998). Overtraining and Recovery: A Conceptual Model. *Sports Med, 26,* 1-16.

Morgan (1980). Test of the champions: the iceberg profile. *Pyschology Today, 6,* 92-108.

Rushall (1990). A tool for measuring stress tolerance in elite athletes. *Journal of Applied Sports Psychology, 2,* 51-66.

Sawka, Burke, Eichner, Maughan, Montain & Stachenfeld (2007). American College of Sports Medicine position stand. Exercise and fluid replacement. *Med Sci Sports Exerc, 39,* 377-390.

Stellingwerff, Boit & Res (2007). Nutritional strategies to optimize training and racing in middle-distance athletes. *J Sports Sci, 25,* 17-28.

Photo & Illustration Credits

Photos Jacket: © fotolia/CHEN, © fotolia/Elena Kalistratova, © fotolia/Daniel Etzold,
© fotolia/karaboux, © fotolia/karaboux, © fotolia/Walter Luger,
© fotolia/Christopher Edwin Nuzzaco, © fotolia, Bakke-Svensson/WTC, Asker Jeukendrup
Cover Design: Sabine Groten
Inside Photos: see individual photos

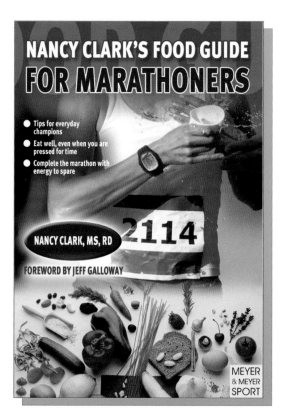

Nancy Clark
Nancy Clark's Food Guide for Marathoners

In Nancy Clark's Food Guide for Marathoners, you'll learn how to eat well, even when you are pressed for time, and how to effectively balance carbohydrates, protein and fat into your diet. After reading Nancy's book you will be able to choose the best snacks for before, during and after long runs, lose weight and have energy to exercise, and even complete an entire marathon with energy to spare!

3rd edition
168 pages, full-color print
27 color photos
Paperback, 6^1/2" x 9^1/4"
ISBN: 9781841262062
$ 16.95 US / $ 29.95 AUS
£ 12.95 UK / € 16.95

The Sports Publisher

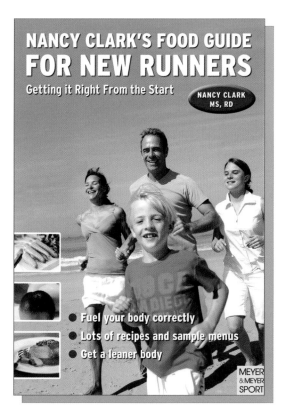

Nancy Clark
Nancy Clark's Food Guide For New Runners

Novice runners are hungry for nutrition advice. What to eat before the run? What about sports drinks? How to lose weight but have enough remaining energy to exercise? Is it normal for runners to get dizzy at the end of a run?

This book will answer all of these questions and many more. The easy-to-read book offers practical tips, debunks nutritional myths, and is a simple "how to" resource for new runners who are eager to learn how to reach their goals with energy to spare.

160 pages, full color print,
15 photos and 53 charts
Paperback, 6^1/2" x 9^1/4"
ISBN: 9781841262628
$ 16.95 US / $ 29.95 AUS
£ 12.95 UK / € 16.95

MEYER & MEYER Sport | www.m-m-sports.com
sales@m-m-sports.com

MEYER
& MEYER
SPORT

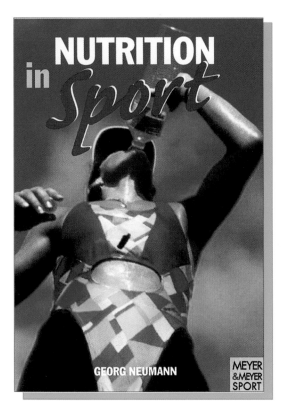

Georg Neumann
Nutrition in Sport

The book makes recommendations for physiologically useful dietary planning before, during and after training in various sports. It also examines risk-prone groups in sports nutrition.
The emphasis is on presenting the latest research on the effects of carbohydrates and proteins and other active substances, such as vitamins and minerals, on perfor-mance train-ing. Particular attention is paid to the intake of food and fluids under special conditions such as training in heat, in the cold and at high altitudes.

224 pages, two-color print
82 full-color pages
31 figures, 51 tables
Paperback, 5 $^3/4$" x 8 $^1/4$"
ISBN: 9781841260037
$ 17.95 US / $ 29.95 AUS
£ 12.95 UK / € 18.90

The Sports Publisher

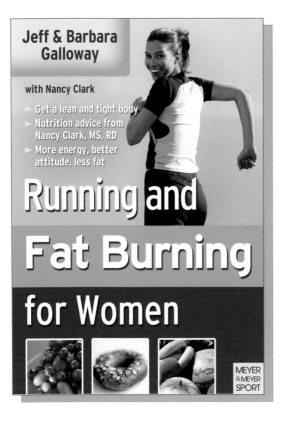

Jeff & Barbara Galloway
Running & Fat Burning for Women

Olympian Jeff Galloway and his wife Barbara offer gentle exertion activity and common-sense eating advice without giving up the wine and chocolate. This easy-to-read book is full of practical tips, successful strategies and meal plans that average women can insert into a busy day. Jeff and Barbara don't just explain the principles in an easy to understand language, they tell you exactly what to eat and how to strategically insert 5-10 minutes of exercise into your day.

2nd Edition
200 pages, full color print,
30 color photos and illustrations
Paperback, 6^1/2" x 9^1/4"
ISBN: 9781841262437
$ 17.95 US / $ 32.95 AUS
£ 14.95 UK / € 16.95

MEYER & MEYER Sport | www.m-m-sports.com
sales@m-m-sports.com